Vestibular Therapy and Rehabilitation

Arne Ernst • Dietmar Basta • Klaus Jahn

Vestibular Therapy and Rehabilitation

Springer

Arne Ernst
MEOCLINIC
Berlin Balance Center
Berlin, Germany

Dietmar Basta
Department of Otolaryngology
Unfallkrankenhaus Berlin
Berlin, Germany

Klaus Jahn
Department of Neurology
Schön Klinik Bad Aibling
Bad Aibling, Germany

ISBN 978-3-031-64317-0 ISBN 978-3-031-64318-7 (eBook)
https://doi.org/10.1007/978-3-031-64318-7

This Springer imprint is published by the registered company Springer Nature Switzerland AG
The registered company address is: Gewerbestrasse 11, 6330 Cham, Switzerland

Preface

This book is an interdisciplinary approach to address a complex field where neurologists, otolaryngologists, geriatricians, physiotherapists, and other medical disciplines are involved. Complaints of dizziness, vertigo, and vestibular disorders have been increased in numbers over the last decades.

The needs of the aging population of the Western world and the technical ability to specifically diagnose vestibular deficits (e.g., by video head impulse, vestibular evoked myogenic potential recordings) have become the main drivers to develop individualized treatment and rehabilitation concepts. They are aimed at targeting the identified underlying disorder responsible for vertigo or dizziness in the individual patient.

Therefore, the whole range of "specific" (e.g., Menière's disease, vestibular migraine), but also "less specific" disease entities (e.g., presbyvestibulopathy, motion sickness) are covered. The general focus of the book is therefore (see the title) "Therapy and Rehabilitation," but not primarily diagnostics.

Vestibular physiotherapy is a well-developed field in the Anglo-American, but also Scandinavian countries, but less represented in the rest of Europe. Thus, we have described some of the vestibular exercises in detail so that the non-specialized therapist might benefit.

Vestibular rehabilitation with technical systems has begun with the introduction of the Balance Master series and related balance platforms about four decades before. This technological field has strongly contributed to new therapies over the last 10 years and is covered in a separate chapter.

We wish this book as a mixture between hands-on style manual and academic tutorial interested readers and therapeutic success for all working in this field!

Berlin, Germany	Arne Ernst
Bad Aibling, Germany	Klaus Jahn
Berlin, Germany	Dietmar Basta
2024	

Acknowledgment

We would like to thank Springer for realizing this project and their professionals working with us, for their openness in finalizing this complicated book, its tables, illustrations, drawings, etc.

Our special thanks goes to Silvy Kellerer for her great help in the preparation of the figures and photographs.

Contents

Part I Basic Principles in Vestibular Therapy

1 Epidemiology and Pathophysiology 3
1.1 Epidemiology of Vestibular Disorders 3
1.2 Habituation and Compensation in Vestibular Disorders 5
1.2.1 Neuronal Mechanisms of Vestibular Rehabilitation 6
1.2.2 Clinical Approaches 7
1.2.3 Adaptation 8
1.2.4 Substitution 9
1.2.5 Habituation 10
References 10

2 General Approaches in Vestibular Disorders 13
2.1 Taking the History, Diagnostics, and Therapy Planning 13
2.1.1 Taking the History in Dizzy Patients 13
2.1.2 Evaluation of the Dizzy Patient by Questionnaires 14
2.1.3 Clinical Examination of the Dizzy Patient 16
2.1.4 Neuro-otological Testing of the Dizzy Patient 17
2.1.5 Neuroimaging of the Dizzy Patient 21
2.1.6 The Therapy Plan for Dizzy Patients 21
2.2 Pharmacological Treatment of Vestibular Disorders 23
2.2.1 Therapeutic Use of Analgesics in Neck Pain with Dizziness 23
2.2.2 Therapeutic Drug Use in Vestibular Disorders 25
2.3 Physical Therapy and Vestibular Rehabilitation in Vestibular Disorders 27
2.3.1 Time Course and Therapy 27
2.3.2 Physical Therapy in Central and Musculoskeletal Disorders 28
2.3.3 Rehabilitation Technology in Vestibular Disorders 35
References 46

Part II Therapy and Rehabilitation of Peripheral and Central Vestibular Disorders

3 Peripheral Vestibular Disorders (Labyrinthine Disorders) 53
3.1 Benign Paroxysmal Positional Vertigo (BPPV). 53
3.1.1 Occurrence and Etiology 53
3.1.2 Diagnostic Procedures 54
3.1.3 Treatment Options 56
3.1.4 Medication 60
3.2 Unilateral Vestibular Loss (UVL) 60
3.2.1 Diagnostic Findings and Differential Diagnosis 60
3.2.2 Time Course and Therapy 61
3.2.3 Risk and Pitfalls 62
3.3 Bilateral Vestibular Loss (BVL). 62
3.3.1 Diagnostic Findings and Differential Diagnosis 62
3.3.2 Time Course and Therapy 63
3.3.3 Risks and Pitfalls 63
3.4 Endolymphatic Hydrops and Menière's Disease (MD). 63
3.4.1 Diagnostic Findings and Differential Diagnosis 63
3.4.2 Time Course and Therapy 64
3.4.3 Risk and Pitfalls 65
3.5 Dehiscence Syndromes of the Semicircular Canals (SCDS/PCDS) 65
3.5.1 Diagnostic Findings and Differential Diagnosis 65
3.5.2 Time Course and Therapy 66
3.5.3 Risks and Pitfalls 67
References. 67

4 Central Vestibular Disorders 71
4.1 Vestibular Schwannoma/Acoustic Neuroma (AN) 71
4.1.1 Diagnostic Findings and Differential Diagnosis 71
4.1.2 Time Course and Therapy 71
4.1.3 Risks and Pitfalls 73
4.2 Vestibular Migraine (VM) 73
4.2.1 Diagnostic Findings and Differential Diagnosis 73
4.2.2 Time Course and Therapy 74
4.2.3 Risks and Pitfalls 74
4.3 Vestibular Paroxysmia (VP). 75
4.3.1 Diagnostic Findings and Differential Diagnosis 75
4.3.2 Time Course and Therapy 76
4.3.3 Risks and Pitfalls 76
4.4 Vestibular Stroke 77
4.4.1 Diagnostic Findings and Differential Diagnosis 77
4.4.2 Time Course and Therapy 77
4.4.3 Risks and Pitfalls 78
References. 78

Part III Therapy and Rehabilitation of Vertigo and Dizziness as Major Symptoms in Different Etiologies

5 Dizziness over the Life-Span 83
5.1 Dizziness in Childhood and Adolescence 83
5.1.1 Taking the History in Children 83
5.1.2 Neuro-otological Examination in Children 84
5.1.3 Differential Diagnosis of Vertigo and Dizziness in Children 85
5.2 Dizziness and Vertigo in the Aging Population 90
5.2.1 Diagnostic Findings and Differential Diagnosis 94
5.2.2 Time Course and Therapy 94
5.2.3 Risks and Pitfalls 95
References 95

6 Dizziness in Cerebral Disorders 99
6.1 Dizziness in Head Trauma and After Concussion 99
6.1.1 Diagnostic Findings and Differential Diagnosis 99
6.1.2 Time Course and Therapy 100
6.1.3 Risk and Pitfalls 101
6.2 Dizziness After Stroke/Cerebral Ischemia 101
6.2.1 Diagnostic Findings and Differential Diagnosis 101
6.2.2 Time Course and Therapy 102
6.2.3 Risks and Pitfalls 102
6.3 Dizziness in Neurodegenerative and Inflammatory Brain Disorders 103
6.3.1 Diagnostic Findings and Differential Diagnosis 103
6.3.2 Time Course and Therapy 103
6.3.3 Risks and Pitfalls 104
6.4 Dizziness and Epilepsy 104
References 104

7 Dizziness in Other Medical Condition 107
7.1 Dizziness in Psychiatric and Psychosomatic Conditions 107
7.1.1 Diagnostic Findings and Differential Diagnosis 107
7.1.2 Time Course and Therapy 107
7.1.3 Risks and Pitfalls 108
7.2 Dizziness with Peripheral Neuropathy 108
7.3 Dizziness After Cochlear Implantation 109
7.3.1 Occurrence and Etiology 109
7.3.2 Prevention 111
7.3.3 Diagnostic Procedures 112
7.3.4 Therapy 112

7.4 Dizziness in Ophthalmology, Cardiology, and Orthopedics 113
7.4.1 Diagnostic Findings and Differential Diagnosis 114
7.4.2 Time Course and Therapy 114
7.4.3 Risks and Pitfalls 115
References. 117

Part IV Other Therapeutic Measures and Specific Interventions in Vestibular Disorders

8 Tai Chi and Other Measures to Improve Gait and Stance Stability 121
References. 122

9 Dietary Measures 123

10 Counselling and Coping for the Dizzy Patient 125

Index. 127

About the Authors

Arne Ernst is board-certified otolaryngologist with a professional training at Tübingen University (Head: Hans Zenner) from 1988 to 1993 and at Hanover Medical School (Head: Thomas Lenarz) from 1993 to 1997. He is Professor and Chairman of the Department of Otolaryngology at UKB Hospital Berlin (Charité Medical School) since 1998 and has developed rehabilitation programs for vestibular disorders, including medical, surgical, and training therapies. He served as Chairman of the Germany Audiology, Neurotology and Otology Group (ADANO) until 2016, is member of several Editorial Boards (e.g., Otology and Neurotology, HNO), and has published on neuro-otology and implantology/otology extensively (240 papers in peer-reviewed journals, 10 textbooks). From 2024 on, he manages the Berlin Balance Center as Clinical Director.

Dietmar Basta holds a Master of Science in Neurobiology and a PhD (Neuroscience) from the Humboldt-University of Berlin, Germany. He was a group leader for hearing research at the University of Potsdam, Germany until 2002. Since 2003, he works at the Department of Otolaryngology at UKB—Charité Medical School, University of Berlin, Germany as the Head of the Center for Applied Medical Technology and as an independent lecturer in Neurophysiology (Privatdozent). His research focus includes diagnostic and treatment methods for vestibular disorders and the mechanisms of hearing loss and prosthetic restitution. He has published more than 150 papers and several textbooks and contributes as a board member to several scientific organizations and international journals.

Klaus Jahn received his Neurology training in Munich at the Technical University (TU; Head: Bastian Conrad) and the Ludwig-Maximilians-University (LMU; Head: Thomas Brandt) in Munich. Between 2006 and 2014 he served as a senior consultant in the same department (Head: Marianne Dieterich). From 2012 to 2014 he was the Director of the German Center for Vertigo and Balance Disorders (DSGZ) at the LMU. He is the Head of the Departments of Neurology and Geriatrics at the Schön Klinik Bad Aibling, Germany since 2015. His clinical and research focus is on balance, gait, vertigo and dizziness, multisensory function, neurology over the life span, and neurorehabilitation. He has published about 240 papers in peer-reviewed journals and is member of several guideline groups in the field.

Abbreviations

ABC	Activities-specific-balance confidence scale
ABR	Auditory brainstem responses (auditory evoked potentials)
AICA	Anterior inferior cerebellar artery
AN	Acoustic neuroma (synonym: vestibular schwannoma)
AVS	Acute vestibular syndrome
BBS	Berg balance scale
BPPV	Benign paroxysmal positional vertigo
BVL	Bilateral vestibular loss
CA	Cerebellar ataxia
CI	Cochlear implant
CNS	Central nervous system
CPA	Cerebello-pontine angle
CROM	Cervical range-of-motion
CSF	Cerebrospinal fluid
CT	Computed tomography
DGI	Dynamic gait index
DHI	Dizziness handicap inventory
DVA	Dynamic visual acuity
EVA	Enlarged vestibular aqueduct
FES	Fall efficacy scale
GCS	Glasgow coma scale
HA	Hearing aid
HINTS	Head impulse/nystagmus/test of skew
HIT	Head impulse test
HL	Hearing loss
IAC	Internal auditory canal
iNFT	Individualized neuro-feedback training
INO	Internuclear ophthalmoplegia
MARS	Mobile app rating scale
MD	Menière's disease
MEMS	Micro-electro-mechanical systems
MRA	Magnetic resonance angiography
MRI	Magnetic resonance tomography
MS	Multiple sclerosis

MSA	Multi-system atrophy
MTBI	Mild traumatic brain injury
nGVS	Noisy galvanic vestibular stimulation
NFT	Neuro feedback training (vibrotactile)
NSAID	Non-steroidal anti-inflammatory drugs
OAE	Otoacoustic emissions
PCDS	Posterior canal dehiscence syndrome
PCS	Post-concussion syndrome
PD	Parkinson's disease
PICA	Posterior inferior cerebellar artery
PMR	Progressive muscular relaxation
PS	Parkinson syndrome
PSP	Progressive supranuclear palsy
PT	Physiotherapy/physical therapy
PTSD	Posttraumatic stress disorder
RCT	Randomized controlled trial
SCC	Semicircular canal
SCDS	Superior canal dehiscence syndrome
SNHL	Sensorineural hearing loss
SRC	Sports-related concussion
SVV	Subjective visual vertical
TENS	Transcutaneous electric nerve stimulation
TEOAE	Transient evoked otoacoustic emissions
TUG	Timed up and go test (Tinetti's test)
UVL	Unilateral vestibular loss (= vestibular neuritis/neuropathy)
c/oVEMP	Cervical/ocular vestibular evoked myogenic potentials
VM	Vestibular migraine
VN	Vestibular neuritis (= UVL)
VOR	Vestibulo-ocular reflex
VP	Vestibular paroxysmia
VRT	Vestibular rehabilitation therapy
VS	Vestibular stroke
VSS	Vertigo symptom scale
WAD	Whiplash-associated disorder

List of Figures

Fig. 1.1 Different types of vestibular symptoms in the general population (From: Neuhauser HK: Epidemiology of dizziness, Handbook of Clinical Neurology 2016) (with permission) 4
Fig. 1.2 (a) Gray-matter signal increases of the right gracile nucleus in patients after UVL. (b) White matter signal increases around the commissural vestibular fibers in the pons projected onto a brainstem template. The results indicate multisensory mechanisms of central vestibular compensation. P = posterior; A = anterior; L = left; R = right (from zu Eulenburg et al. 2010) 7
Fig. 1.3 Principles of vestibular compensation 8
Fig. 2.1 Taking the patient's history with key questions 14
Fig. 2.2 Diagnostic approach according to the patient's history 14
Fig. 2.3 Clinical examination of the dizzy patient with an acute vestibular syndrome (AVS). Clinical findings in AVS 17
Fig. 2.4 Clinical examination of the dizzy patient with chronic dizziness 17
Fig. 2.5 Domains of ocular motor function and their testing 19
Fig. 2.6 Cover test in heterophoria and heterotropia 20
Fig. 2.7 Overview of all components of a specialized VRT program 22
Fig. 2.8 Individual therapy planning and follow-up 22
Fig. 2.9 (Physiological) cervical range of motion (CROM) (a) lateroflexion—clavicular/eye line; (b) ventral/dorsal flexion—plane of occlusion; (c) rotation—sagittal plane) 24
Fig. 2.10 PT in central vestibular disorders (PCS: post-concussion syndrome; TBI: traumatic brain injury; others (MS, mal de debarquement syndrome; cerebellar ataxia) are dealt with VRT techniques separately (see Chaps. 6 and 7) 28
Fig. 2.11 Exercises for gait disorders 29
Fig. 2.12 Exercises for balance disorders 32
Fig. 2.13 Exercises for acute vertigo/dizziness 36

Fig. 2.14 Example of an auditory feedback device application (SwayStar®) 41
Fig. 2.15 Example of a visual feedback device (Balance Quest®) 42
Fig. 2.16 Example of a galvanic feedback device (PoNS®) 44
Fig. 2.17 Example of a vibrotactile feedback device application (Vertiguard®). The arrows indicate vibratory stimulators which are activated by the main unit. The main unit is connected "head-down" on the same belt for a better usability by the patient. 46
Fig. 3.1 Dix-Hallpike maneuver to detect BPPV(p). (a) Fast positioning of the head in reclination (20°) with the tested ear directed to the ground. (b) Observation of nystagmus with Frenzel's goggles for at least 1 min. (from Ernst and Basta (2016), with courtesy of the Georg Thieme Verlag KG) 55
Fig. 3.2 Epley's (a) and Semont's (b) maneuver to treat p-BPPV (from Parnes et al. 2003, with courtesy of the Canadian Medical Association) 58
Fig. 3.3 Yacovino maneuver to treat a-BPPV (from Albernaz et al. (2019), with courtesy of Springer Nature). 59
Fig. 3.4 Gufoni's maneuver to treat h-BPPV (from Albernaz et al. (2019), with courtesy of Springer Nature). 59
Fig. 3.5 Diagnostic/therapeutic procedure in patients with UVL (PT Physiotherapist, VRT Vestibular rehabilitation therapy) 61
Fig. 3.6 International consensus (ICON) on the treatment of Menière's disease (Nevoux et al. 2018) (ITC Intratympanic therapy with dexamethasone—DXM, ITG Intratympanic gentamicin, ELSS Endolymphatic shunt surgery, VN Vestibular neurectomy, CI Cochlear implantation), comment: VN is usually replaced nowadays by surgical occlusion of the lateral SCC (Charpiot et al. 2010). 64
Fig. 3.7 SCDS at different locations of the SCC (A: normal; B1–3: different locations at the eminentia arcuata; C: SCDS by the superior petrous sinus) 66
Fig. 4.1 Acoustic neuroma (VN) with intra-/extrameatal extension (MRI scan). 72
Fig. 4.2 Neurorehabilitation approach in AN-patients after therapy (microsurgical resection/radiotherapy) with/without pre-hab (see text) (superior/inferior VN—vestibular nerve; VRT—vestibular rehabilitation; PT—physical therapy) 72
Fig. 4.3 Susceptible area of the vestibular-cochlear nerve (asterisk: AICA loop) at the root entry zone and other cranial nerves where vascular cross compression causes paroxysmal symptoms. 75

Fig. 4.4 Lesion distribution in stroke patients with the leading symptoms vertigo, dizziness, or double vision (Zwergal et al. 2020) 78
Fig. 5.1 Frequency distribution among dizzy children (Jahn et al. 2015b) 85
Fig. 5.2 Dizziness and imbalance in elderly age 91
Fig. 6.1 Upon concussion/impact, a pressure wave passes from the CSF space to the inner ear through its connecting pathways (cochlear/vestibular aqueduct) and impairs the cochlear/vestibular receptor cells 100
Fig. 6.2 Wallenberg's syndrome: Clinical presentation and site of lesion 101
Fig. 7.1 Pathophysiology of functional dizziness and anxiety-related symptoms (Wuehr et al. 2013) 108
Fig. 7.2 Saccular membrane distortion upon cochlear implant electrode insertion. (**A**) Distorted saccular membrane. (**B**) Saccular sensory epithelium, arrows indicate pathological movements of the saccular membrane (after Tien and Linthicum Jr. 2002) 111
Fig. 7.3 PT in neuro-orthopedic disorders with acute onset (e.g., whiplash injury, post-surgery of the cervical spine) (MRI: magnetic resonance imaging of the cervical spine; CROM: determination of the cervical range of motion) 114
Fig. 7.4 Home exercises for the cervical/ thoracal spine 115

List of Tables

Table 1.1 Prevalence and incidence of vertigo in the general population (Neuhauser 2016) . . . 5
Table 2.1 Relevant aspects to test with ocular motor examination . . . 19
Table 2.2 Non-opioid analgesics, dosage regime, major side effects, and indications . . . 25
Table 2.3 Pharmacotherapy of vestibular disorders . . . 26
Table 5.1 Taking the history in dizzy children and adolescents . . . 84
Table 5.2 Therapy of peripheral vestibular disorders in children . . . 86
Table 5.3 Therapy of central vestibular disorders in children . . . 87
Table 5.4 Common causes of vertigo and dizziness in the elderly . . . 91
Table 5.5 Common causes of gait abnormalities in the elderly . . . 92
Table 5.6 Domains of balance impairments in elderly subjects . . . 92
Table 7.1 Overview about the percentage of function loss in specific vestibular sensors upon cochlear implantation in relation to the surgical electrode insertion approach (c = insertion via cochleostomy, rw = round window insertion) . . . 110
Table 8.1 The ten principles of Tai Chi Chuan exercises (https://kung-fu.co.za/articles/10-principles-of-tai-chi-chuan) . . . 122

Part I

Basic Principles in Vestibular Therapy

Different kinds of compensation are the physiological principles which underlay all those intrinsic processes where the vestibular system starts after being challenged by vestibular disease, acute disorder, etc. It is important for all those involved in therapy that there is a time pattern which should be used by intervention to improve and speed-up those mechanisms. Some approaches are more effective for the treatment of a specific vestibular dysfunction than others. This chapter will give an overview about the basic principles. In addition, apart from vestibular rehabilitation interventions, in some cases, drug prescription can be helpful.

Epidemiology and Pathophysiology 1

1.1 Epidemiology of Vestibular Disorders

"Dizziness" is the second most common complaint when patients see a general practitioner (GP) in the Western world (second after headache). In Germany, about 25% of the population complains of dizziness at least once a year (Lempert and Neuhauser 2009). The 12-months' incidence of "dizziness" is 3.1% in Germany, but only 1.4% for original vestibular disorders, both with a female dominance (Neuhauser 2009). Vestibular disorders have a high sociomedical relevance as they are accompanied by longer periods of being unable to work (41% vs. 15% in "dizziness"), social inactivity (40% vs. 10% in "dizziness") and tend to lead to somatization (19% vs. 10% in "dizziness"). This inevitably leads to the question of a correct, full neurological diagnostic workup of patients which is limited by capacity. Taking the history of the patients is very important to reveal correlations between migraine (14% lifetime prevalence) and vestibular disorders (specifically: benign paroxysmal positional vertigo—BPPV, Meniere's disease—MD) (von Brevern and Neuhauser 2011), depression and vestibular disorders (Neuhauser et al. 2005), as well as cardiovascular and vestibular disorders (Neuhauser et al. 2005) (Fig. 1.1).

> The most frequent vestibular disorder (by diagnosis) is BPPV which is increasingly prevalent in the 60+ population (3.4% for 12 months) with a cumulative re-occurence rate of 50% in the first year after onset. The second most frequent vestibular disorder is vestibular migraine (VM).

VM has emerged after reclassification of migraine-related disorders by the International Headache society (IHS) and the Barany Society (Lempert et al. 2012). VM has a lifetime prevalence of 0.98% with female dominance, particularly after the menopause (Neuhauser et al. 2006). The third most frequent vestibular disorder

A. Ernst et al., *Vestibular Therapy and Rehabilitation*,
https://doi.org/10.1007/978-3-031-64318-7_1

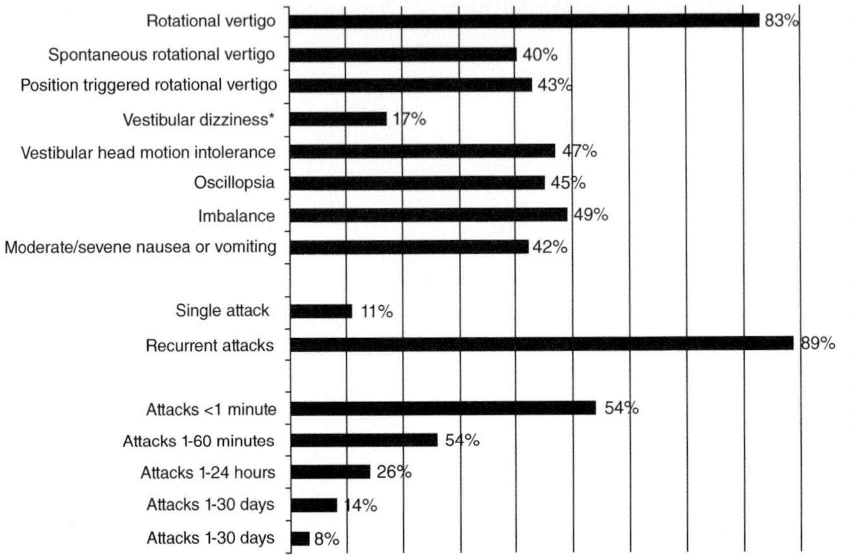

Fig. 1.1 Different types of vestibular symptoms in the general population (From: Neuhauser HK: Epidemiology of dizziness, Handbook of Clinical Neurology 2016) (with permission)

is UVL with a 12-month incidence of 24/100,000 (only hospitalized patients included) (Neuhauser and Lempert 2009). MD is assumed to occur with an annual incidence of 15/100,000 (at medium ages 40–60 years), a usually unilateral disorder which is frequently overdiagnosed (Neuhauser and Lempert 2009). One-third of all MD patients suffers from bilateral occurrence and/or VM in parallel (Neuhauser and Lempert 2009).

A general problem of epidemiological data for "dizziness" and/or vestibular disorders is that they are based on different diagnostic criteria, thus diagnostic quality (either questionnaire/interview or screening tests) differs. If a specialized balance center is involved, data become highly selective and not more representative for the whole population (e.g., Strupp and Brandt 2008).

As with the aging of all sensory systems, the vestibular system also declines in structure and functionality so that vestibular disorders ("presbyvestibulopathy") are threefold more frequent in the 70+ population compared to younger adults (Neuhauser et al. 2005).

US data suggest that 69% of the 70+ population have a prevalent balance deficit (compared to 63% for hearing loss—HL) (Zuniga et al. 2012) (Table 1.1).

Table 1.1 Prevalence and incidence of vertigo in the general population (Neuhauser 2016)

% of the adult population (95% CI)						
	Women	(95% CI)	Men	(95% CI)	Total	(95% CI)
Dizziness[a] of moderate or severe intensity						
Incidence (1-year)	4.0	(3.2–5.0)	2.3	(1.6–3.1)	3.1	(2.6–3.8)
Prevalence (1-year)	28.9	(26.8–31.1)	16.7	(15.0–18.6)	22.9	(21.5–24.3)
Prevalence (lifetime)	35.9	(33.7–38.3)	22.6	(20.6–24.7)	29.3	(27.8–30.9)
Dizziness[a] leading to sick leave, medical consultation, or interruption of daily activities						
Incidence (1-year)	2.6	(2.0–3.5)	1.4	(0.9–2.1)	2.0	(1.6–2.5)
Prevalence (lifetime)	24.0	(22.0–26.1)	12.8	(11.3–14.5)	18.5	(17.2–19.8)
Vestibular vertigo						
Incidence (1-year)	1.9	(1.4–2.7)	0.8	(0.4–1.3)	1.4	(1.0–1.8)
Prevalence (1-year)	7.1	(6.0–8.4)	2.6	(1.9–3.5)	4.9	(4.2–5.7)
Prevalence (lifetime)	10.3	(9.0–11.8)	4.3	(3.4–5.4)	7.4	(6.5–8.3)

Based on data from Neuhauser et al. (2005, 2009)
CI Confidence interval
[a]Dizziness including vertigo

The structural degeneration of the peripheral vestibular receptors is based on a decline in sensory (vestibular hair) cells (Rauch et al. 2001) and follows a certain pattern, i.e., the semicircular canals (SCC) are followed by the saccule and, finally, the utricle in functional loss (Agrawal et al. 2012). Those elderly with marked vestibular deficits fall more often and more severely compared to age matched non-fallers (Liston et al. 2014). Comorbidities which play a role in the progression and clinical picture of presbyvestibulopathy include cognitive and psychiatric impairment and limited visuospatial abilities due to brain changes (Bigelow and Agrawal 2015).

1.2 Habituation and Compensation in Vestibular Disorders

The loss or reduction of afferent information in the ascending vestibular pathway (e.g., in acute vestibular syndrome—AVS) induces a strong and long-lasting disorganization of the vestibular system. Such pathophysiological changes induce static and dynamic vestibular deficits which in turn cause postural, perceptual, and ocular motor syndromes (Lacour 2006). The postural syndrome involves inclination of the head and body toward the affected side as well as incapacity to stabilize the posture while moving, especially for rotational movement of the body/head toward the affected side. The perceptual syndrome comprises vertigo with deviation of the subjective visual vertical and spatial disorientation. The ocular motor syndrome includes spontaneous nystagmus, vertical misalignment (skew deviation), and ocular cyclotorsion (ocular tilt reaction) (Halmagyi et al. 1991; Lopez et al. 2005).

Mainly cerebral plasticity contributes to the recovery of balance (Lacour 2006). Adjustments of internal models and weighting of sensory inputs are likely at least as important as the readjustment of reflexes by the modulation of network activity in the brainstem (bilateral vestibular nuclei) or within cerebellar structures. An internal model (also called Kalman filter) weights the degree to which a sensory input affects the ongoing state of postural control. The internal model is adjusted by experience and continuously incorporates changes of sensory inputs. This provides a method of adjusting for the salience and reliability of sensory streams. In this regard, vestibular rehabilitation adjusts the internal model by teaching the patient to compensate for unreliable sensory streams.

1.2.1 Neuronal Mechanisms of Vestibular Rehabilitation

The knowledge about specific neuronal mechanisms of vestibular compensation is limited. One important central nervous correlate of vestibular compensation is the recovery of resting activity in the vestibular nuclei (VN). This is not mainly related to the contralateral afferent input (Cartwright et al. 1999) in UVL, since bilateral vestibular deafferentation is also followed by a recovery of resting activity in both VNs (Ris and Godaux 1998). The regeneration of VN resting activity seems to be based on different mechanisms. Changes in the efficacy of synaptic inputs from the spinal cord is either based on axonal sprouting or increased transmitter release (Vidal et al. 1998), changes in postsynaptic receptors, and changes in the intrinsic properties of VN neurons (Peusner et al. 1998). In addition, results suggested that changes in glial cell distribution may be causally involved in the recovery of resting activity in the VN (Campos Torres et al. 1999). Astrogenesis and interestingly also neurogenesis occur after deafferentation in the VN. This was shown to contribute highly to vestibular compensation (Dutheil et al. 2009).

Even if there is an approximate correlation between the recovery of resting activity in the VN and the compensation of the vestibular symptoms, considerable compensation of some symptoms should occur before resting activity is regenerated in some areas of the VN (Ris et al. 1997). Therefore, further mechanisms should be considered to explain the vestibular compensation in peripheral vestibular loss. A significant increase of gray-matter volume in the insular vestibular cortex and superior temporal gyrus could be correlated with improved clinically assessed vestibular deficits and self-assessed vestibular impairment (Helmchen et al. 2009). Significant increases in gray-matter volume upon vestibular compensation were also observed in the bilateral hippocampus, visual cortices, and the cerebellum (Hong et al. 2014). White matter increases in the commissural fibers as a direct consequence of an increased inter-nuclei vestibular crosstalk of the medial vestibular nuclei in the vestibular system. To regain postural stability during vestibular rehabilitation, a shift to the somatosensory system due to an elevated processing of proprioceptive information in the right gracile nucleus could be observed (Fig. 1.2). Furthermore, an

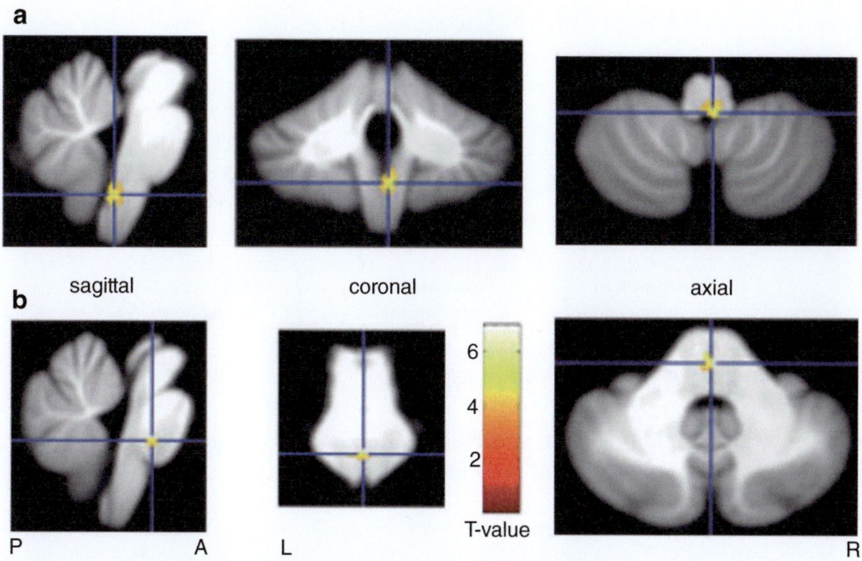

Fig. 1.2 (**a**) Gray-matter signal increases of the right gracile nucleus in patients after UVL. (**b**) White matter signal increases around the commissural vestibular fibers in the pons projected onto a brainstem template. The results indicate multisensory mechanisms of central vestibular compensation. P = posterior; A = anterior; L = left; R = right (from zu Eulenburg et al. 2010)

increased importance of visual motion process during vestibular rehabilitation is related to an increase of white matter around the middle temporal MT/V5 (zu Eulenburg et al. 2010). All these results indicate a multisensory contribution to vestibular rehabilitation.

However, it is open so far how vestibular compensation occur when the end-organ is intact, but the VN cortical stream is interrupted (e.g., due to a thalamic stroke). There is some evidence that multiple plastic processes at various sites in the brain—including cerebellum, entorhinal cortex, and hippocampus—are involved in vestibular compensation of central lesions (Dutia 2010). Animal studies indicated mechanisms of vestibular compensation upon a thalamic lesion by augmented metabolic activation in the cerebellum, mainly contralateral, and in contralateral subcortical structures such as superior colliculus, while diminished activation was observed in ipsilateral visual, entorhinal, and somatosensory cortices. These results indicate compensatory processes in the non-affected sensory systems of the intact brain side (Reuss et al. 2020).

1.2.2 Clinical Approaches

The time-course of vestibular rehabilitation (VRT) varies in a wide range and depends on many different factors. In general, static deficits mostly recover within days while a dynamic deficit recovers frequently in months and even do not to

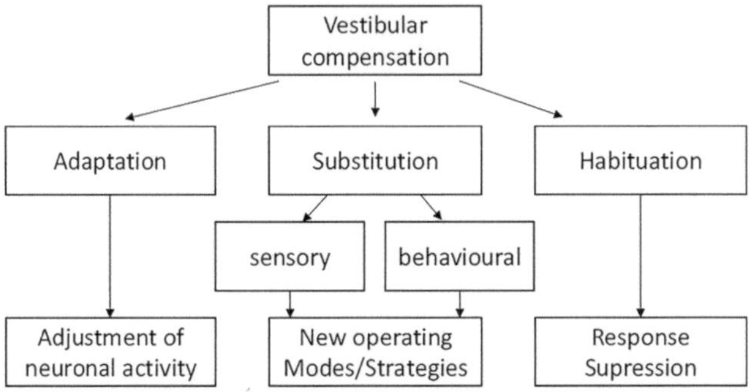

Fig. 1.3 Principles of vestibular compensation

recover totally when looking at vestibular testing in detail (Borel et al. 2004; Borel et al. 2002; Lacour et al. 2009; Lopez et al. 2007).

VRT by cerebral plasticity is based on three main mechanisms of central compensation (Fig. 1.3). These are adaptation, substitution, and habituation (Lacour 2006).

1.2.3 Adaptation

The adaptation provides the regulation of the neuronal activities mainly of the vestibulo-ocular reflex (VOR). The VOR physiologically enables the stabilization of a visual target onto the fovea and consists in a displacement of the eye whose movement is exactly the opposite of the head movement. The quotient between the head and the eye movement (gain) is equal to unity in the physiological condition. After a loss of vestibular afferent information, the gain is reduced and oscillopsia occurs. The adaptation increases the gain of the VOR to stabilize vision. Adaptive plasticity for peripheral vestibular lesions is remarkably powerful and even able to reverse the VOR (Gonshor and Jones 1976). The cerebellar flocculus is a key structure where such adaptive changes occur since the gain of the VOR is adjusted and maintained by this area. Lesions of the flocculus reduce the possibility to adapt to disorders, which reduce or increase the gain of the VOR. Some exercise in vestibular rehabilitation can dramatically support the adaptation. Especially, the fixation training may reduce the intensity of the nystagmus and may explain a fast recovery (Huy and Charfi 2008). The grade of the gain reduction and the time frame between the vestibular loss and the start of the rehabilitation seem to be predictive for the rehabilitation benefit. Patients with a gain below 0.2 are frequently not able to compensate by adaptation (Lacour et al. 2021). VRT should start as early as possible since the efficiency declines after 30 days dramatically (Lacour et al. 2020). However, a dysfunction of the VOR persists far after the resolution of the dizziness without complains (Lopez et al. 2005), suggesting adaptation is not the primary mechanism of vestibular compensation.

Adaptation exercises consist of performing head movements while keeping a target in focus. A typical setup is that a patient is asked to look at a target in front of him and move his head side to side while keeping the target in focus. The exercises should be gradually enhanced by pushing the speed to a level just before the target falls off-focus. As function improves, the exercise can be advanced to moving the target opposite to head movement. For a faster improvement, the exercise can be performed in various positions (i.e., sitting, standing, lying, walking), distances, and speeds (Dye et al. 2013).

1.2.4 Substitution

The substitution is based on different mechanisms initiated by the central nervous system in the sensorial, behavioral, and cognitive domains. This is related to an increased contribution of the proprioceptive, visual, and probably auditory inputs for the equilibrium. The weighting of sensory cues is individual-specific. A re-weighting illustrates the substitution phenomenon. The visual sensorial substitution, on the one hand, is particularly of interest in the process of VRT, as the visual inputs have the priority of all information. On the other hand, visual dependence explains why patients rely on vision to compensate their deficit even if this could have a negative impact on a successful vestibular compensation. The behavioral substitution is an avoidance strategy that limits the movements to diminish the vertigo-related feeling. This "immobilization" is not recommended since conversely early mobilization of patients accelerates and improves the amelioration of posture by compensating the slow phase of the nystagmus. This compensation is indicated by covert saccades (saccades during the head movement) in the video head impulse test. The cognitive substitution corresponds to the anticipation of movements by the patients. A patient would anticipate, e.g., a situation of head rotation by a rotation of the whole trunk and head (instead of the head alone).

Substitution exercises are designed for the improvement of the visual and somatosensory inputs, using exercises that challenge balance without vision, with disturbed vision, or on uneven/soft surfaces. These balance exercises can enhance the use of the vestibular input and should be performed to challenge both static and dynamic balance. However, in case of severe damage to the vestibular function, exercises without visual inputs are not indicated because increasing visual and proprioceptive inputs is mandatory for a successful compensation by sensory substitution. Hence, the rehabilitation program should be highly individualized and related to daily-life conditions since there is a high degree of context dependency to the repair of peripheral vestibular lesions. For example, a patient who was trained to stabilize gaze on a target with the head in a fixed position may not be able to do so when making the same with head movements (Baker et al. 1987). Similarly, when the VOR is trained using head movements of low frequency, no training effect is seen at high frequencies (Godaux et al. 1983).

1.2.5 Habituation

Compensation by habituation is mainly based on teaching the patients to avoid responding to a perturbation. Repetitions of cycle of rotational movements reduce the VOR and diminish oscillopsia. Visual perturbation with rotational light stimuli reduces the visual dependence. This phenomenon is linked to the loss of postsynaptic potentials in neurons exposed to a repeated electrical stimulation (Tee and Chee 2005).

Habituation exercises aimed to increase the thresholds of the clinical response by the repetition of the stimulus. Habituation exercises are the focus of vestibular rehabilitation in patients with benign paroxysmal position vertigo after particle repositioning maneuvers. It has been shown that combining positional maneuvers with vestibular rehabilitation improve outcomes (Chang et al. 2008). During the habituation training, it is always crucial to identify the condition that induces a clinical sign and to repeat them with the therapist at increasing intensity.

References

Agrawal Y, Zuniga MG, Davalos-Bichara M et al (2012) Decline in semicircular canal and otolith function with age. Otol Neurotol 33(5):832–839. https://doi.org/10.1097/MAO.0b013e3182545061

Baker J, Wickland C, Peterson B (1987) Dependence of cat vestibulo-ocular reflex direction adaptation on animal orientation during adaptation and rotation in darkness. Brain Res 408(1–2):339–343. https://doi.org/10.1016/0006-8993(87)90401-x

Bigelow RT, Agrawal Y (2015) Vestibular involvement in cognition: visuospatial ability, attention, executive function, and memory. J Vestib Res 25(2):73–89. https://doi.org/10.3233/VES-150544

Borel L, Harlay F, Magnan J et al (2002) Deficits and recovery of head and trunk orientation and stabilization after unilateral vestibular loss. Brain 125(Pt 4):880–894. https://doi.org/10.1093/brain/awf085

Borel L, Harlay F, Lopez C et al (2004) Walking performance of vestibular-defective patients before and after unilateral vestibular neurotomy. Behav Brain Res 150(1–2):191–200. https://doi.org/10.1016/S0166-4328(03)00257-2

von Brevern M, Neuhauser H (2011) Epidemiological evidence for a link between vertigo and migraine. J Vestib Res 21(6):299–304. https://doi.org/10.3233/VES-2011-0423

Campos Torres A, Vidal PP, de Waele C (1999) Evidence for a microglial reaction within the vestibular and cochlear nuclei following inner ear lesion in the rat. Neuroscience 92(4):1475–1490. https://doi.org/10.1016/s0306-4522(99)00078-0

Cartwright AD, Curthoys IS, Gilchrist DP (1999) Testable predictions from realistic neural network simulations of vestibular compensation: integrating the behavioural and physiological data. Biol Cybern 81(1):73–87. https://doi.org/10.1007/s004220050545

Chang WC, Yang YR, Hsu LC et al (2008) Balance improvement in patients with benign paroxysmal positional vertigo. Clin Rehabil 22(4):338–347. https://doi.org/10.1177/0269215507082741

Dutheil S, Brezun JM, Leonard J et al (2009) Neurogenesis and astrogenesis contribution to recovery of vestibular functions in the adult cat following unilateral vestibular neurectomy: cellular and behavioral evidence. Neuroscience 164(4):1444–1456. https://doi.org/10.1016/j.neuroscience.2009.09.048

Dutia MB (2010) Mechanisms of vestibular compensation: recent advances. Curr Opin Otolaryngol Head Neck Surg 18(5):420–424. https://doi.org/10.1097/MOO.0b013e32833de71f

Dye DC, Eakman AM, Bolton KM (2013) Assessing the validity of the dynamic gait index in a balance disorders clinic: an application of Rasch analysis. Phys Ther 93(6):809–818. https://doi.org/10.2522/ptj.20120163

Godaux E, Halleux J, Gobert C (1983) Adaptive change of the vestibulo-ocular reflex in the cat: the effects of a long-term frequency-selective procedure. Exp Brain Res 49(1):28–34. https://doi.org/10.1007/BF00235538

Gonshor A, Jones GM (1976) Extreme vestibulo-ocular adaptation induced by prolonged optical reversal of vision. J Physiol 256(2):381–414. https://doi.org/10.1113/jphysiol.1976.sp011330

Halmagyi GM, Curthoys IS, Brandt T et al (1991) Ocular tilt reaction: clinical sign of vestibular lesion. Acta Otolaryngol Suppl 481:47–50. https://doi.org/10.3109/00016489109131342

Helmchen C, Klinkenstein J, Machner B et al (2009) Structural changes in the human brain following vestibular neuritis indicate central vestibular compensation. Ann N Y Acad Sci 1164:104–115. https://doi.org/10.1111/j.1749-6632.2008.03745.x

Hong SK, Kim JH, Kim HJ et al (2014) Changes in the gray matter volume during compensation after vestibular neuritis: a longitudinal VBM study. Restor Neurol Neurosci 32(5):663–673. https://doi.org/10.3233/RNN-140405

Huy PT, Charfi S (2008) Physiological bases and practices in vestibular rehabilitation. Ann Otolaryngol Chir Cervicofac 125(5):273–281. https://doi.org/10.1016/j.aorl.2008.06.003

Lacour M (2006) Restoration of vestibular function: basic aspects and practical advances for rehabilitation. Curr Med Res Opin 22(9):1651–1659. https://doi.org/10.1185/030079906X115694

Lacour M, Dutheil S, Tighilet B et al (2009) Tell me your vestibular deficit, and i'll tell you how you'll compensate. Ann N Y Acad Sci 1164:268–278. https://doi.org/10.1111/j.1749-6632.2008.03731.x

Lacour M, Tardivet L, Thiry A (2020) Rehabilitation of dynamic visual acuity in patients with unilateral vestibular hypofunction: earlier is better. Eur Arch Otorhinolaryngol 277(1):103–113. https://doi.org/10.1007/s00405-019-05690-4

Lacour M, Thiry A, Tardivet L (2021) Two conditions to fully recover dynamic canal function in unilateral peripheral vestibular hypofunction patients. J Vestib Res. https://doi.org/10.3233/VES-201557

Lempert T, Neuhauser H (2009) Epidemiology of vertigo, migraine and vestibular migraine. J Neurol 256(3):333–338. https://doi.org/10.1007/s00415-009-0149-2

Lempert T, Olesen J, Furman J et al (2012) Vestibular migraine: diagnostic criteria. J Vestib Res 22(4):167–172. https://doi.org/10.3233/VES-2012-0453

Liston MB, Bamiou DE, Martin F et al (2014) Peripheral vestibular dysfunction is prevalent in older adults experiencing multiple non-syncopal falls versus age-matched non-fallers: a pilot study. Age Ageing 43(1):38–43. https://doi.org/10.1093/ageing/aft129

Lopez C, Borel L, Magnan J et al (2005) Torsional optokinetic nystagmus after unilateral vestibular loss: asymmetry and compensation. Brain 128(Pt 7):1511–1524. https://doi.org/10.1093/brain/awh504

Lopez C, Lacour M, Ahmadi AE et al (2007) Changes of visual vertical perception: a long-term sign of unilateral and bilateral vestibular loss. Neuropsychologia 45(9):2025–2037. https://doi.org/10.1016/j.neuropsychologia.2007.02.004

Neuhauser HK (2009) Epidemiology of dizziness and vertigo. Nervenarzt. 80(8):887–94. https://doi.org/10.1007/s00115-009-2738-9. PMID: 19626307 Review. German

Neuhauser HK (2016) The epidemiology of dizziness and vertigo. Handb Clin Neurol 137:67–82. https://doi.org/10.1016/B978-0-444-63437-5.00005-4

Neuhauser HK, Lempert T (2009) Vertigo: epidemiologic aspects. Semin Neurol 29(5):473–481. https://doi.org/10.1055/s-0029-1241043. Epub 2009 Oct 15. PMID: 19834858 Review

Neuhauser HK, von Brevern M, Radtke A et al (2005) Epidemiology of vestibular vertigo: a neurotologic survey of the general population. Neurology 65(6):898–904. https://doi.org/10.1212/01.wnl.0000175987.59991.3d

Neuhauser HK, Radtke A, von Brevern M et al (2006) Migrainous vertigo: prevalence and impact on quality of life. Neurology 67(6):1028–1033. https://doi.org/10.1212/01.wnl.0000237539.09942.06

Peusner KD, Gamkrelidze G, Giaume C (1998) Potassium currents and excitability in second-order auditory and vestibular neurons. J Neurosci Res 53(5):511–520. https://doi.org/10.1002/(SICI)1097-4547(19980901)53:5<511::AID-JNR1>3.0.CO;2-C

Rauch SD, Velazquez-Villasenor L, Dimitri PS et al (2001) Decreasing hair cell counts in aging humans. Ann N Y Acad Sci 942:220–227. https://doi.org/10.1111/j.1749-6632.2001.tb03748.x

Reuss S, Siebrecht E, Stier U et al (2020) Modeling vestibular compensation: neural plasticity upon thalamic lesion. Front Neurol 11:441. https://doi.org/10.3389/fneur.2020.00441

Ris L, Godaux E (1998) Neuronal activity in the vestibular nuclei after contralateral or bilateral labyrinthectomy in the alert guinea pig. J Neurophysiol 80(5):2352–2367. https://doi.org/10.1152/jn.1998.80.5.2352

Ris L, Capron B, de Waele C et al (1997) Dissociations between behavioural recovery and restoration of vestibular activity in the unilabyrinthectomized guinea-pig. J Physiol 500(Pt 2):509–522. https://doi.org/10.1113/jphysiol.1997.sp022037

Strupp M, Brandt T (2008) Diagnosis and treatment of vertigo and dizziness. Deutsches Arzteblatt Int 105(10):173–180. https://doi.org/10.3238/arztebl.2008.0173

Tee LH, Chee NW (2005) Vestibular rehabilitation therapy for the dizzy patient. Ann Acad Med Singap 34(4):289–294

Vidal PP, de Waele C, Vibert N et al (1998) Vestibular compensation revisited. Otolaryngol Head Neck Surg 119(1):34–42. https://doi.org/10.1016/S0194-5998(98)70171-8

zu Eulenburg P, Stoeter P, Dieterich M (2010) Voxel-based morphometry depicts central compensation after vestibular neuritis. Ann Neurol 68(2):241–249. https://doi.org/10.1002/ana.22063

Zuniga MG, Dinkes RE, Davalos-Bichara M et al (2012) Association between hearing loss and saccular dysfunction in older individuals. Otol Neurotol 33(9):1586–1592. https://doi.org/10.1097/MAO.0b013e31826bedbc

General Approaches in Vestibular Disorders

2

2.1 Taking the History, Diagnostics, and Therapy Planning

When approaching the dizzy patient, it comes to the different medical disciplines involved. Apart from audiologists and physiotherapists, GPs, neurologists, ENTs, and specialized neuro-otologists all see those patients. The following chapter should guide the professionals through diagnostics/differential diagnosis and help to introduce therapy planning in brief. Neurotological test procedures will not be described in detail.

2.1.1 Taking the History in Dizzy Patients

Taking the history of the patient gives decisive hints on the pathogenesis/time-course and specific underlying disorder(s).

The following points should be addressed (Figs. 2.1 and 2.2):

- Begin and duration of the vestibular symptoms (sudden onset, stepwise increase, intermittent, only seconds), was it the first time?
- Exogenous/endogenous influences/temporal pattern (accidents, head trauma, surgery before, influences by body position/movement, physical/psychological exhaustion, other medical disorders, e.g., stroke, cardiac arrhythmia, new glasses, viral infection, menstrual cycle, new drug intake)
- Specific character of the vestibular symptom (spinning/rotational/attack-like, increased body sway, lateropulsion, fall (tendency), lift feeling, dizziness/unsteadiness, "empty head "feeling)
- Accompanying, non-vestibular symptoms (hearing loss/tinnitus, visual symptoms, e.g., blurred vision, scotoma, hemianopia; falls, loss of consciousness, headache, aura, vomiting/nausea, anxiety)

A. Ernst et al., *Vestibular Therapy and Rehabilitation*, https://doi.org/10.1007/978-3-031-64318-7_2

Questions to ask a patient with vestibular disorder	*Current functional status*
1. Do you experience spells of vertigo (a sense of spinning)? If yes, how long do these spells last?	1. Are you independent in self-cure activities?
2. When was the last time the vertigo occurred? 3. Is the vertigo spontaneous, induced by motion induced by position changes?	2. Can you drive: • In the daytime? • In the nighttime?
4. Do you experience a sense of being off-balance (disequilibrium)? If yes, is the feeling of being off-balance constant, spontaneous, induced by motion, induced by position changes, worse with fatigue, worse in the dark, worse outside, worse on uneven surfaces?	3. Are you working? If yes, occupation: ________ 4. Are you on medical disability?
5. Does the feeling of being off-balance occur when you are lying down sitting, standing or walking?	5. Can you perform all your normal parenting activities?
6. Do you stumble, stagger or side-step while walking? 7. Do you drift to one side while you walk? If yes to which side do you drift? 8. At what time of day do you feel best? ________ worst? ________ 9. How many times per day do you experience symptoms?	6. Do you have difficulty: • Watching TV? • Reading? • Being in stores or malls? • Being in traffic? • Using a computer?
10. Do you have hearing problems? 11. Do you have visual problems?	7. Do you have difficulty walking up and down ramps, stairs, walking on grass?
12. Have you been in an accident (e.g. motor vehicle)? 13. What medications do you take? 14. Do you live alone? 15. Do you have stairs in your home? 16. Do you smoke? If yes, please indicate how much per day. 17. Do you drink alcohol? If yes, please indicate how much.	

Fig. 2.1 Taking the patient's history with key questions

ENT ↓
- Otomicroscopy
- Endoscopy of pharynx, nose
- Balance screening tests
- Audiological testing (if required)

Neurology ↓
- Cranial nerves (I-XII) testing
- motor function testing
- sensitivity (deep paths) testing
- coordination testing

↘ ↙
- neuroimaging (HR-CT, MRA)

Fig. 2.2 Diagnostic approach according to the patient's history

- Previous medical disorders (chronic otitis media, sinusitis, diabetes, whiplash injury, neurological disorders of the brain parenchyma, ophthalmic/cardiovascular disorder, psychiatric illness)
- Drug intake (sedatives, psychopharmacological/cardiovascular drugs)

2.1.2 Evaluation of the Dizzy Patient by Questionnaires

Questionnaires are helpful to better assess the patient's complaints under specific medical perspectives. The symptoms (and subjective complaints) on the one hand have to be correlated with the objective findings of neurotological testing on the other, but there is more. How much anxiety or fear of falling is in the patient's description (ABC, FES, VSS)? How much is the mobility/gait performance impaired (DGI, TUG)? How is the static/dynamic/functional balance performance of geriatric patients, e.g., after hospitalization/acute stroke (BBS)? Can we follow-up the training effects on functional, physical, emotional level (DHI)?

One test is not sufficient to answer all questions. There is no one-test-fits-all, and each test design has its limitations. However, the point scores can help to quantify the success rate of VRT, sometimes they also have a good predictive value (e.g., for falls).

2.1.2.1 ABC

The *A*ctivities-specific *B*alance *C*onfidence Scale (ABC) was developed as psychometric tool for seniors to detect the loss of balance confidence in highly functioning seniors with more specific situations-specificity than FES of the items, also used to plan therapy (Powell and Myers 1995).

https://doi.org/10.23668/psycharchives.401

2.1.2.2 BBS

The *B*erg *B*alance *S*cale (BBS) was developed to assess geriatric patients, their balance stability (static, dynamic, functional, interplay of the vestibular subsystems) and to assess their fall risk. It is inappropriate to evaluate gait capabilities (Berg and Norman 1996). It correlates well with the Barthel's index and TUG. It has a high predictive value for falls (Muir et al., 2010).

https://www.researchgate.net/publication/234059090_Berg-Balance-Scale-deutsche_Version_Berg-Balance-Scale-German_Version

2.1.2.3 DHI

The *D*izziness *H*andicap *I*nventory (DHI) is a comprehensive questionnaire aiming at the "functional" (everyday activity), "physical" (physical activity/performance), and "emotional" (psychosomatic condition) performance (as subscale, with a point scoring system) of the patients. The total, but also the subscores are well suited to follow-up training/VRT effects.

https://geriatrictoolkit.missouri.edu/vest/Dizziness-Handicap-Inventory.pdf

2.1.2.4 DGI

The *D*ynamic *G*ait *I*ndex (DGI) is aimed at assessing the impact of peripheral/central vestibular disorders in geriatric patients (but also in stroke, Parkinson's, etc.) on movement/gait. It is highly relevant for everyday activities, but less specific/sensitive than other tests (Whitney et al. 2004).

https://www.researchgate.net/publication/250879086_Functional_Gait_Assessment_-Functional_Gait_Assessment

2.1.2.5 FES

The *F*all *E*fficacy *S*cale (FES) was developed by Tinetti et al. (1990) as an instrument to measure fear of falling in mainly community-dwelling elderly population. The study was based on the operational definition of fear of falling, which is "low perceived self-efficacy at avoiding falls during essential, non-hazardous activities of daily living."

https://www.researchgate.net/publication/6887640_The_German_version_of_the_Falls_Efficacy_Scale-International_Version_FES-I

2.1.2.6 TUG

The *T*imed-*u*p-and-go *t*est (TUG) is an easy-to-perform test (getting up from a chair, walking 3 m, turn around, go back, and sit down) (Tinetti et al. 2000) so that it is frequently used as a screening tool to evaluate the individual physical capabilities of elderly. It has a high variability of the test results and can therefore only be used to screen/differentiate geriatric patients (mobile/immobile/higher fall risk).

https://www.verywellhealth.com/the-timed-up-and-go-test-2696072

2.1.2.7 VSS

The *V*ertigo *S*ymptom *S*cale (VSS) (Yardley et al. 1992) can help to differentiate organic vs. non-organic (functional) vertigo so that it should be particularly used as diagnostic screening tool, when the patients complain of chronic dizziness.

https://www.vumc.org/balance-lab/sites/vumc.org.balance-lab/files/public_files/Dizziness%20Symptom%20Profile%20-%20Vanderbilt%20UMC.pdf

2.1.3 Clinical Examination of the Dizzy Patient

The clinical examination of the dizzy patient should follow some algorithms to differentiate the types of vestibular disorders (Fig. 2.3). The clinical assessments have to include ENT- and neurology-aspects of vestibular function.

2.1.3.1 ENT

The examination should include otoscopy (microscopy) to search for signs of acute or chronic inflammation (tympanic membrane) and/or efflorescence in/around the external ear canal (e.g., zoster oticus). An endoscopic examination of the nose (sinusitis?) and pharynx/larynx (paresis? inflammation?) should follow.

2.1.3.2 Neurology

Most dizzy patients cannot differentiate if their complaints come from vestibular problems, from deficits in other sensory channels, or just from erroneous perception of physiological regulations (functional dizziness). The neurological examination therefore has to include the following (Jahn et al. 2015):

- Testing of the ocular motor (see below), visual (visual acuity), and vestibular systems (head impulses, positioning maneuvers)
- Testing of function of peripheral nerves (peripheral neuropathy: tendon reflexes, sense of vibration, proprioception)

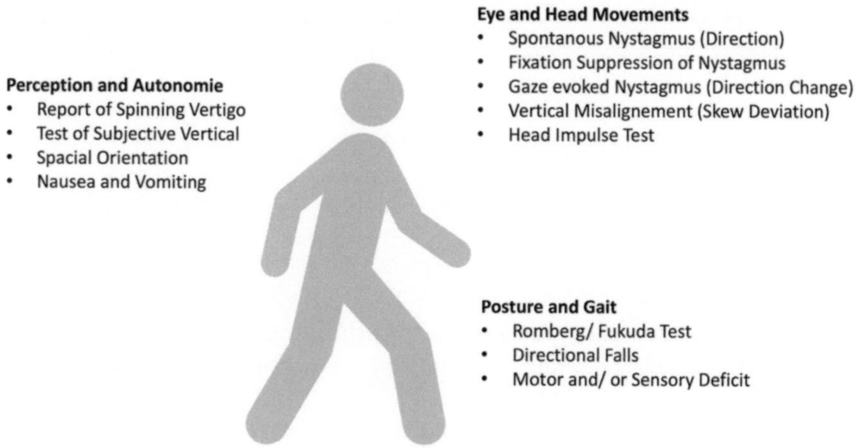

Fig. 2.3 Clinical examination of the dizzy patient with an acute vestibular syndrome (AVS). Clinical findings in AVS

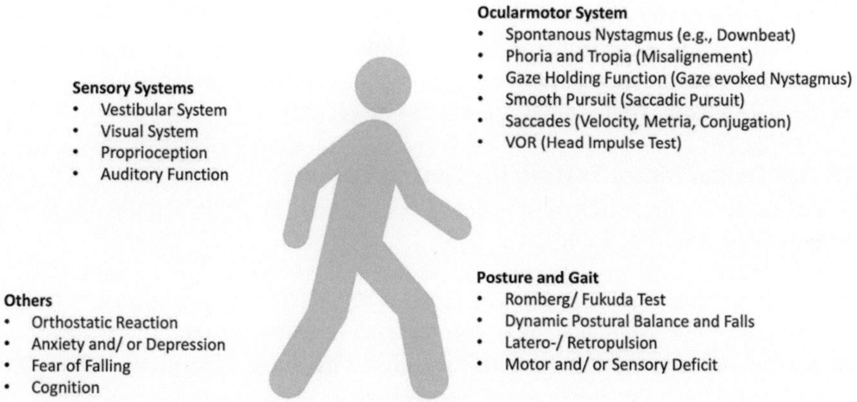

Fig. 2.4 Clinical examination of the dizzy patient with chronic dizziness

- Testing of stance and gait under different conditions (Romberg test, tandem stance with eyes open and closed, walking at different velocities and under dual-task)
- Testing of central coordination (cerebellar function) and motor function (spasticity with increased tendon reflexes) (Fig. 2.4)

2.1.4 Neuro-otological Testing of the Dizzy Patient

2.1.4.1 Screening Tests

Screening tests should be used as bedside ones or by first-line caretakers (GP/emergency physician/paramedic).

Frenzel goggles are helpful to screen for the existence of a spontaneous (e.g., in UVL), a positional (e.g., in BPPV in Dix-Hallpike position), or head-shake nystagmus (e.g., UVL in remission).

Gait and stance tests (Romberg/standing on foam with eyes open/eyes closed) have low specificity (about 30%), but can indicate a vestibular deficit (e.g., lateropulsion to the affected side, increased sway in central vestibular deficits).

The head impulse test (HIT) can be done at the bedside to differentiate between a UVL and acute stroke affecting the VN (PICA-infarction; it is often normal in the latter, despite AVS).

2.1.4.2 Neuro-otological Testing (Incl. Audiological Testing)

Neuro-otological testing is required when a specific peripheral or central vestibular deficit should be diagnosed.

The semicircular canals (SCC) should be tested first by the head impulse test (HIT) for each spatial plane (fast phase of the VOR) to detect (acute) pathology. Caloric examination (of the lateral SCC) is helpful in chronic dizziness and to judge the extent of compensation after an acute UVL (slow phase of the VOR). HIT and caloric testing do not always match.

Otolith testing by c/oVEMPs (sacculus/utricle) or by other means (subjective visual vertical—SVV, eccentric rotation) is important for complex or long-standing vestibular disorders. The extent of residual otolith input (e.g., after resection of vestibular schwannoma) determines the success of VRT.

2.1.4.3 Ocular Motor Testing for Central Deficits

The figure shows the different domains of ocular motor function and the respective examinations (Fig. 2.5; Table 2.1).

> It is worth learning how to examine the ocular motor system. It provides a look into the brain and is more sensitive than MRI scans (Kim et al. 2022). A complete clinical examination of the ocular motor systems will take only 1–2 min with some experience.

It is important not just to test eye movements in general, but the different functional systems in separation (Leigh and Zee 2006). This is also a prerequisite for effective therapy, as combined eye-head movements are an important part of vestibular rehabilitation (Meldrum and Jahn 2019).

First, the **spontaneous position** of the eyes should be observed. Manifest misalignments with larger amplitudes will be visible by asymmetric corneal reflexes. Mild misalignments, however, will only become evident with cover tests (Fig. 2.6). Heterophoria (latent deviations) and heterotropia (manifest deviations) must be distinguished.

Smooth pursuit eye movements are tested for the horizontal and vertical directions with velocities of up to 100°/s. Testing should start with low velocities and

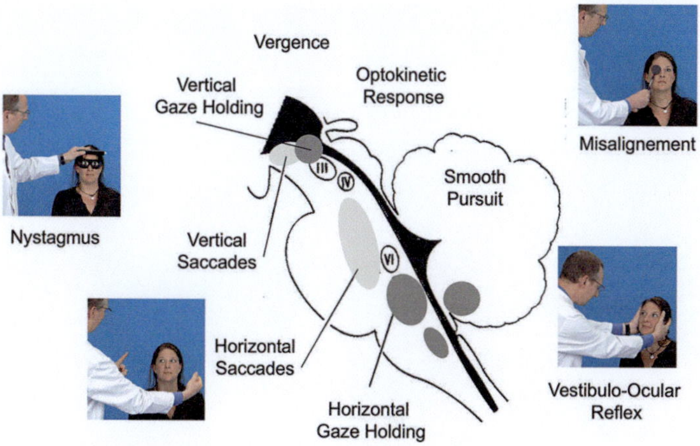

Fig. 2.5 Domains of ocular motor function and their testing

Table 2.1 Relevant aspects to test with ocular motor examination

Test for	Comment	Test
Heterophoria, Heterotropia	Latent (phoria) or manifest (tropia) misalignment of the eyes	Cover test
Skew deviation	Vertical misalignment (Tropia) of the eyes; part of the ocular tilt reaction; sensitive brainstem sign	Cover test
Ocular tilt reaction	Mostly central sign (sensitive brainstem sign) with skew deviation, ocular tilt, ocular torsion, tilted perception of verticality	Cover test, Test for Subjective Visual Vertical (SVV), Observation of head tilt
Smooth pursuit deficits and disturbed suppression of VOR	Smooth pursuit eye movements (<100°/s) and the ability to suppress the VOR use the same networks, involving the cerebellum	Follow a target of low velocity (e.g., finger of the examiner) in horizontal and vertical directions, without head movements (smooth pursuit) or combined with head movement (suppression of VOR)
Gaze holding function	A deficit results in gaze evoked nystagmus; network centers are in the lower brainstem for horizontal and in the upper brainstem for vertical eye movements	Gaze holding in eccentric positions (e.g., 20°) for the horizontal and for the vertical plane
Saccades	Network centers are in the lower brainstem for horizontal and in the upper brainstem for vertical eye movements	Jumps to eccentric gaze positions for the horizontal and for the vertical plane
Nystagmus	Spontaneous nystagmus in primary position in acute vestibular syndrome (suppressed by fixation, horizontal and torsional) or with central lesions/degeneration (e.g., downbeat nystagmus)	Primary position gaze with and without fixation of a target (e.g., with Frenzel goggles); eccentric positions to distinguish from gaze evoked nystagmus

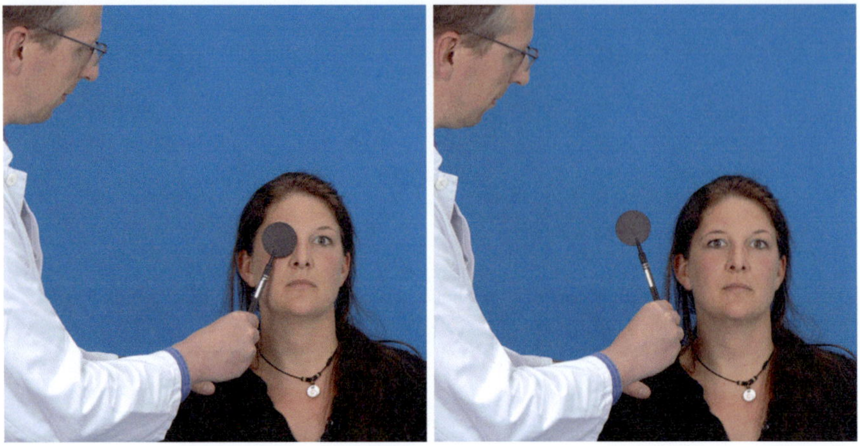

Fig. 2.6 Cover test in heterophoria and heterotropia

increase velocity until pursuit becomes saccadic, which will be the case at some point. Cave: Elderly people often show some saccadic pursuit due to minor dysfunction in the network (e.g., with mild vascular encephalopathy). Younger subjects can show saccadic pursuit in vestibular migraine (Dieterich and Brandt 1999) but also with brain diseases (e.g., multiple sclerosis). Saccadic pursuit is also a typical finding in cerebellar disorders. Saccadic pursuit often goes along with disturbed suppression of the VOR which uses the same brain network.

Gaze-evoked nystagmus can be observed at eccentric eye positions. 30° lateral gaze and 20° up–/downward gaze are sufficient for testing. End-point gaze-evoked nystagmus is not a specific sign of pathology. Gaze-evoked nystagmus in general is most often observed as side effect of drugs and medication (e.g., carbamazepine, phenytoin). Horizontal gaze-evoked nystagmus can be a sign of lesions in the lower brainstem (leaky integrator for horizontal eye movements). Vertical gaze-evoked nystagmus points to an integrator lesion in the upper brainstem (mesencephalon).

Saccades are tested for the horizontal and vertical planes by observing gaze jumps to eccentric points. Velocity, precision, and conjugation of both eyes are looked at. Normal saccades are metric (exact to the point), fast (>300°/s), and conjugated. In patients, hypermetric saccades are always pathological and point to a cerebellar lesion. Slow saccades are observed with lesions of the respective centers on pontine (horizontal) and mesencephalic (vertical) brainstem level. A slowing of saccades is also observed with neurodegeneration (e.g., Progressive Supranuclear Palsy = PSP). Complete and severe lesions of the centers cause complete gaze palsy for the horizontal or vertical plane. Disconjugation of both eyes is observed in internuclear ophthalmoplegia (INO), which is most often seen in multiple sclerosis (lesion of the medial longitudinal fascicle = MLF).

2.1.4.4 Audiological Testing

When patients also complain of hearing loss (HL) and/or tinnitus, they should be examined as well by a pure-tone audiogram (PTA) to differentiate low-frequency

HL (e.g., in MD), from high-frequency HL (e.g., in AN) or severe HL (e.g., as in labyrinthine infarction). Objective audiological tests (TEOAE = Transient Evoked Otoacoustic Emissions for the inner ear, i.e., the integrity of the outer hair cells) and ABR (Auditory Brainstem Responses, to detect central auditory processing disorders) are suggested.

2.1.5 Neuroimaging of the Dizzy Patient

High resolution computer tomography (HR-CT) of the temporal bones should be done in suspected inflammatory or other lesions (e.g., malformations). The most important indications are suspected middle ear/mastoid infections, SCDS, EVA, and cochleo-vestibular malformations.

MRI/MRA investigations focus on the internal auditory canal (= IAC, e.g., in AN), the cerebellopontine angle (= CPA, e.g., in neurovascular conflicts), and the brain parenchyma to identify pathology. Any recurrent acute vestibular disorder should be investigated at least once by MRI/MRA.

2.1.6 The Therapy Plan for Dizzy Patients

> Coping and counselling the dizzy patient are essential to prepare the ground for a full cooperation, a positive motivation, to prevent anxiety/somatization/personal frustration based on any vestibular disorder and to build up trust and self-confidence as the basis for a successful therapy.

2.1.6.1 Counselling the Dizzy Patient

This should be done in a timely manner, starting with the explanation of the underlying vestibular disorder, its time-course, and the therapeutic steps the patient should follow (Fig. 2.7). You should address:

- Type of disorder, natural course (compensation, habituation), etiology
- Comorbidity as related to the vestibular disorder (e.g., arterial hypertension, dehydration)
- Therapy plan and medical measures (incl. Medication, PT/VRT)
- What can the patient do (e.g., sports, healthy lifestyle, home exercises)!
- Active anti-anxiety management (encouraging the patient, reinforce motivation).

2.1.6.2 Timing the Therapy Measures

The therapy plan for each patient is based on the underlying vestibular disorder and should be customized/individualized. While peripheral vestibular disorders (e.g., UVL) are primarily treated by VRT, central ones should be dealt with also by

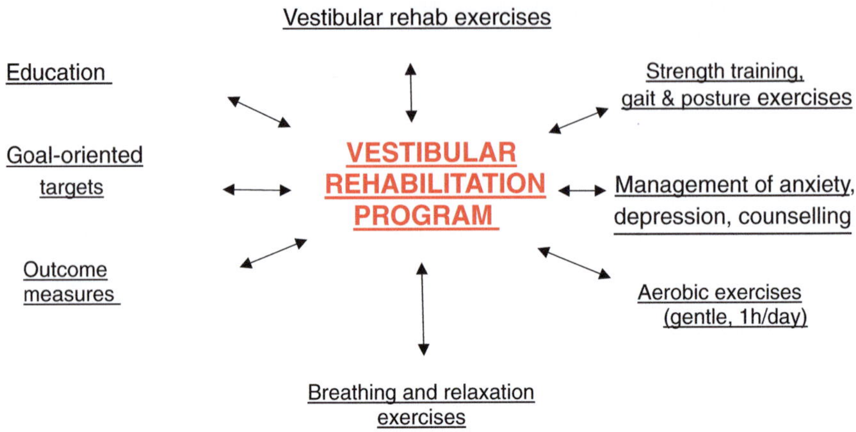

Fig. 2.7 Overview of all components of a specialized VRT program

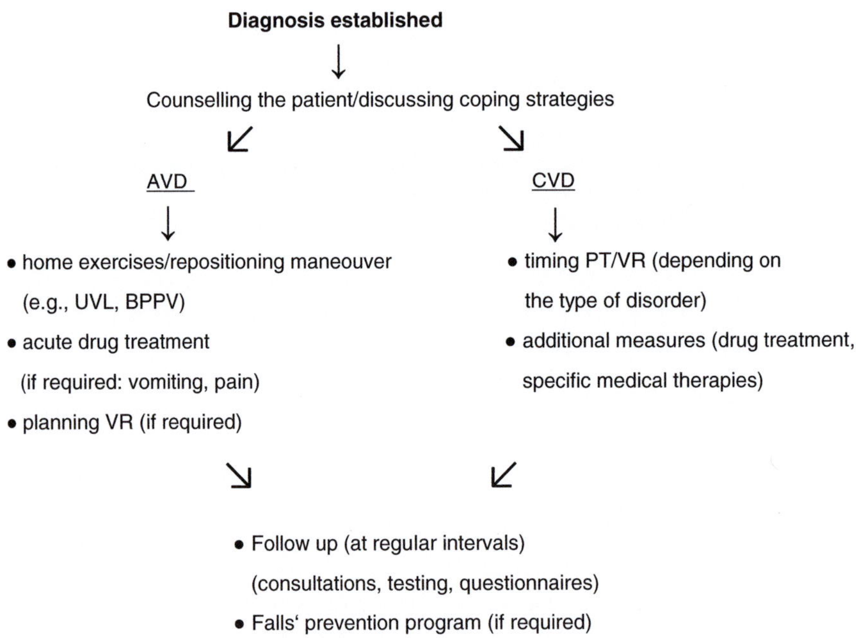

Fig. 2.8 Individual therapy planning and follow-up

PT. Apart from this, the individual medical/physical condition and therapeutic progress should be taken into account (advancement of exercises may be "too fast," which leads to frustration and failure) to tailor the individual therapy plan (Fig. 2.8).

The dizzy patient should be followed-up at regular intervals (on an individual basis) until VRT/PT and the overall therapeutic progress have plateaued and the patient has reached a level of normalized lifestyle. This will not always be possible in a reasonable period-of-time (e.g., after stroke), but a regular follow-up at certain intervals (e.g., 6 weeks/3 months within the first year after the onset) should be done by consultation/neurotological testing, including the questionnaires (see above) and a focus on the possible sequalae of an acute vestibular disorder (e.g., falls). Possibly, a specialized falls'prevention program can be added after the end of the initial VRT/PT program.

2.1.6.3 Follow-Up of the Dizzy Patient

2.2 Pharmacological Treatment of Vestibular Disorders

Pharmacological therapeutic options are widely used to treat dizzy patients. Evidence, however, is still insufficient for several indications. Nonetheless drug treatment is helpful in many clinical situations (Zwergal et al. 2019; Lemos and Manto 2022).

2.2.1 Therapeutic Use of Analgesics in Neck Pain with Dizziness

Analgesics are primarily used in acute/chronic pain conditions of the head and neck and the cervical spine, in particular. The following major pain-related disorders affect any vestibular rehabilitation approach since physiological/pathophysiological correlations interfere with the VRT protocols (for details, see below):

- Cervical/head trauma/pain (blunt trauma/spinal concussion, whiplash trauma, post-surgical pain/scars—e.g., after discectomy-, cervical spine stenosis, fibromyalgia)
- Cervicogenic headache
- (classical) Migraine and tension headache

2.2.1.1 Diagnostic Findings and Differential Diagnosis

The most prominent finding is the neck pain intensity as related to the (limited) cervical range of motion (CROM). The pain can be acute after the trauma or chronic which is the case in many dizzy patients. There are different ways of evaluation: manual diagnostics, measuring CROM or subjective rating (e.g., Numerical Pain Rating Scale or Neck Disability Index; Langevin et al.,

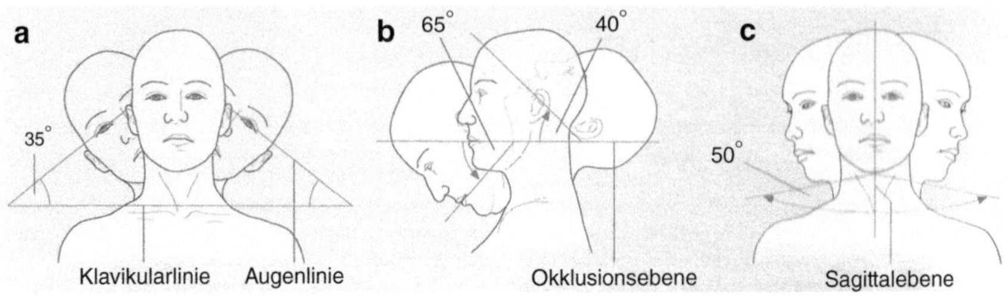

Fig. 2.9 (Physiological) cervical range of motion (CROM) (**a**) lateroflexion—clavicular/eye line; (**b**) ventral/dorsal flexion—plane of occlusion; (**c**) rotation—sagittal plane)

2019) (Fig. 2.9). Usually, they have none or minor pathological neuroimaging findings, but pain and related health problems are based on a chronic inflammatory response of the overstretched cervical muscles with accompanying cervical joints.

When the CROM is decreased (e.g., after hypothermia or physical overload), cervicogenic headache can occur. This can also trigger a pre-existing classical migraine and/or tension-type headache. In patients with blockade (reversible joint dysfunction) at C0/C1, this is most prominent. Many patients with cervical pain complain of a feeling of dizziness, particularly when closing their eyes. This is related to the (relative) stiffening of the postural muscles along the spine (postural imbalance) and can be recorded as an increase in trunk sway by mobile posturography (Rossi-Izquierdo et al. 2016), a finding likely in many MTBI (Mild Traumatic Brain Injury) patients (Table 2.2).

The patient should be counselled that VRT is only helpful when the pain is under full control, i.e., any intervention should be possibly performed pain-free. Pain limits the effectiveness of PT/VRT since it blocks a processing of vestibular and other information at the level of the brainstem and at higher CNS levels (for review see Feller et al. 2020). In whiplash patients, VRT can decrease the self-perceived handicap and increase postural control (Ekvall Hansson et al. 2006).

2.2.1.2 Time Course and Therapy

The acute neck patient is usually not seen/diagnosed/treated primarily in a VRT unit. We therefore refer to the literature for the acute phase (advocating a combination of manual therapy-analgesics and exercises, for review, see Hidalgo et al. 2017). The chronic pain patient, however, is often diagnosed and treated for the self-perceived dizziness. The followings aspects must be considered when preparing a VRT protocol:

- Analgesics should be applied until the pain cessates, primarily NSAIDs since they do not interfere with the CNS (Table 2.3). This should be supported by manual therapy and home exercises (see Fig. 7.4).

Table 2.2 Non-opioid analgesics, dosage regime, major side effects, and indications

Non-opioid analgesics	Daily (max) dosage	Major side-effects	Indications
NSAID			
Ibuprofen	3 × 600 mg	GIT toxicity, renal insufficiency, cardiac failure, arterial hypertension	Short-term intake in peripheral pain (and inflammation), combine with PPI (if necessary)
Diclofenac	2 × 75 mg		
Selective COX2-inhibitors			
Etoricoxib	Once 90 mg	Renal insufficiency, cardiovascular disorders as contraindication, bronchial spasms	Very effective in GIT toxicity by NSAID
Celecoxib	2 × 200 mg		
Antipyretic analgesics			
Paracetamol	3 × 1000 mg	Hepatotoxicity	Peripheral pain, no GIT tox.
Metamizole	4 × 1 g	Hypotension agranulocytosis	Spasmolytic, no GIT tox.
Others			
Pregabalin	4 × 75 mg	Reduction of renal clearance, nausea, sleepiness	Neuropathic pain (pain-induced depression)

NSAID non-steroidal anti-inflammatory drug, *COX* cyclooxygenase, *GIT* gastro-intestinal trac, *PPI* proton pump inhibitors

- If neuropathic pain (e.g., after spinal concussion) is prevalent, other approaches (e.g., therapeutic local anesthetics at trigger points, TENS systems, acupuncture, PMR) should be applied before pregabalin is considered since this drug is known to cause dizziness/vertigo as one of the more common side effects.
- Fibromyalgia patients pose a complex challenge and should be treated together with their primary (pain specialist/rheumatologist) caretaker.

2.2.1.3 Risks and Pitfalls

Pain and traumatic brain injury patients are the greatest challenge to any VRT program. The best outcome in those conditions with VRT can be achieved when a complex rehabilitation protocol (incl. analgesic procedures, manual therapy, coping, and counselling) can be applied. VRT per se does not change neck pain or CROM (Hansson et al. 2013). Accompanying medical conditions (e.g., depression, anxiety) should be treated accordingly (see Chap. 7).

2.2.2 Therapeutic Drug Use in Vestibular Disorders

The table summarizes drug use in the treatment of different vestibular disorders (Table 2.3). Symptomatic treatment in the acute vestibular syndrome is indicated whenever a patient suffers from acute vertigo, nausea, vomiting, and falls (Jahn

Table 2.3 Pharmacotherapy of vestibular disorders

Kind of use/indication/ clinical reasoning	Substance group/specific drugs and dosages	Comments
Suppression of acute vestibular symptoms (vertigo, nausea, vomiting)	Dimenhydrinate 50–150 mg (p.o./i.v./supp.); Benzodiazepines, e.g., Lorazepam 1 mg (s.l.)	Short term use in acute vestibular syndrome (1–3 days); sedation as major side effect
Acute treatment of anxiety in vestibular disorders	Benzodiazepines, e.g., Lorazepam 1 mg (s.l.)	Rare and short-term use; combination with psychotherapy is essential
Prophylactic treatment in vestibular migraine (VM)	A number of substances are available and are used in analogy to headache migraine, e.g.,: Metoprolol 50–100 mg/day, Topiramate 25–50 mg/day, Amitriptylin 10–30 mg/day	Substance should be chosen based on additional therapeutic effects (e.g., lowering blood pressure with Metoprolol) and the likelihood of side effects (e.g., cognitive problems with Topiramate)
Prophylactic treatment in Menière's Disease (MD)	Betahistine 60–220 mg/d; combination with Selegiline increases bio-availability	In general, well tolerated, but mediocre evidence
Prophylactic treatment in Vestibular Paroxysmia (VP)	Sodium-channel blocking drugs, e.g., Carbamazepine 200–400 mg/ day, Lamotrigine 25–100 mg/day, Lacosamide 20–200 mg/day, Oxcarbazepine 150–300 mg/ day	Response to treatment is part of the diagnostic criteria; Lamotrigine and Lacosamide are better tolerated on the long run
Prophylactic treatment in Episodic Ataxia (Type 2; EA)	4-Aminopyridine 5–20 mg/ day, Acetazolamide 250–500 mg/ day	Genetic disorder (autosomal dominant) that requires long-term treatment
Functional Dizziness	SSRI, e.g., Citalopram 10 mg/day	Combined with psychotherapy
Acute Unilateral Vestibulopathy/ Vestibular Neuritis	Methylprednisolone in different schemes for 3–8 days	Combination with symptomatic treatment (vestibular suppression) for the first 1–3 days
Motion Sickness/ Kinetosis	Dimenhydrinate 20–50 mg every 6 h in symptomatic situations (e.g., driving in a bus or mobile home)	Short-term use, sometimes indicated in children
Downbeat- (Upbeat-) Nystagmus	4-Aminopyridine 5–20 mg/ day	Off-label, individual therapy trial

2016). It should not be given in the long run. Drug therapy to specifically address the etiology of symptoms is possible for vestibular paroxysmia and episodic ataxia (Strupp et al. 2011, 2019). Prophylactic treatment to avoid further attacks or at least reduce their frequency is useful in vestibular migraine and Menière's disease (Zwergal et al. 2019; Feil et al. 2018; Lemos and Manto 2022).

Pharmacological treatment of vestibular disorders is often helpful. It should, however, be specific for the diagnosis and only given for the time required (e.g., a few days for symptomatic treatment of the acute vestibular syndrome). Chronic vestibular disorders (e.g., VM or MD) are an exception and need long-term treatment since this treatment includes pharmacological prophylaxis of the attacks in episodic vestibular disorders.

2.3 Physical Therapy and Vestibular Rehabilitation in Vestibular Disorders

Principles of physical therapy are essential in the rehabilitation of peripheral, but also central vestibular disorders (Whitney and Sparto 2011; Hall et al. 2016, 2022).

After an acute onset of vertigo/dizziness, the patients with peripheral vestibular loss undergo a phase of static compensation (i.e., reestablishment of static gaze stability) within the first 5–10 days where they should be carefully mobilized so that they can move on their own. Thereafter (phase of dynamic compensation), specific vestibular rehabilitation exercises (e.g., Cawthorne-Cooksey exercises and its current modifications) should be applied so that an individualized VRT approach aimed at the specific deficit (e.g., the lateral SCC or the otolith/macular organs) is achieved.

More complex are the therapies *for central vestibular disorders* (e.g., after ischemic stroke, cerebral hemorrhage, head trauma) because other limiting disabilities (e.g., hemiplegia, motor dysfunction, reduced skin sensitivity, anopia) of the sensory, motor, and cognitive domains have to be considered. In general, PT or physiotherapy (usually done in small groups) requires in those patients a neurorehabilitation team with specialized professionals (physiotherapists, occupational therapists, sports therapists, etc.) to cover the highly variably aspects of the different vestibular disorders and to individualize the therapy options ("tailoring the approach") (Whitney and Sparto, 2011; Hall et al. 2022).

2.3.1 Time Course and Therapy

Apart from BPPV (see Chap. 3), unilateral vestibular loss (UVL) is the most relevant, acute, peripheral vestibular disorder. The patients complain of spinning vertigo, nausea, and vomiting in the acute ("critical") phase. Cerebellar and/or brainstem (PICA) infarction is the most important differential diagnosis (and can be distinguished by HINTS/neuroimaging). UVL symptoms recover completely in about 2/3 of the patients within 3 weeks to 3 months (i.e., central compensation, VOR adaptation, structural restoration). In the first 5–10 days, mobilization by a/with a physiotherapist and self-exercises (if possible) are helpful.

2.3.2 Physical Therapy in Central and Musculoskeletal Disorders

Central vestibular disorders are usually sequelae of ischemic, hemorrhagic, or traumatic events that affect not only the vestibular nuclei (brainstem) or the central vestibular network. The patients can be mobilized (e.g., balance and gait training, strengthening, coordination, proprioception, endurance, and flexibility exercises) (Brown et al., 2006, Ekvall Hansson et al., 2006) when they are able to move (Fig. 2.10). This is aimed at improving general health and physical conditioning (with motor skills and normalized gait in particular) and can last up to years. It is helpful in all phases of neurorehabilitation (Veerbeek et al. 2014) and is aimed at the major deficits to activate habituation, if possible. Patients with impaired function of the vestibular nuclei (e.g., by brainstem infarction) need similar treatment as BVL patients.

Physical therapy as classical musculoskeletal therapy (whether manual medicine or osteopathy) is important in patients with pain and/or other posttraumatic disorders (e.g., after head trauma and/or whiplash). They require a passive/active mobilization of the affected head and neck region (muscles, joints, ligaments) to make VRT possible (Fig. 7.4). In addition, a home training program is advised (Figs. 2.11, 2.12, 2.13). Medication is often additionally helpful (see Chap. 2). Other types of central vestibular disorders (e.g., MS, cerebellar ataxia, vestibular migraine, Mal de Debarquement syndrome) require specific VRT measures (see Chap. 4).

Acute onset (e.g, PCS, TBI, stroke)

↓

Neurotological/neurological diagnostics

↓

Active/passive mobilization, strengthening, coordination, proprioception, endurance exercises (improving motor skills/normalize gait)

↙ ↘

Home training for postural muscles | specific VR exercises

Fig. 2.10 PT in central vestibular disorders (PCS: post-concussion syndrome; TBI: traumatic brain injury; others (MS, mal de debarquement syndrome; cerebellar ataxia) are dealt with VRT techniques separately (see Chaps. 6 and 7)

1. Walking while moving the head

(walk 3-5 minutes with and without a target fixation, change head position every three steps):

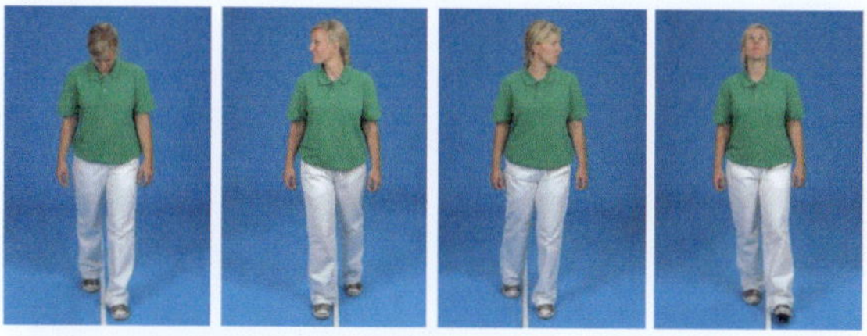

2. Speeding up and slowing down

(walk at normal pace in the first part of the way, accelerate the walking speed to maximum in the second part and slowdown in the last third, repeat all up to 2 min):

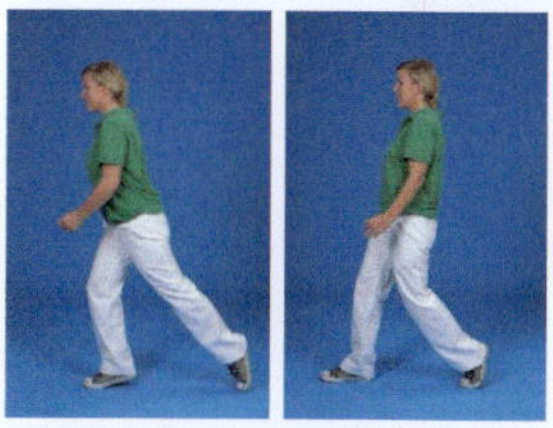

3. Stepping over obstacles

(walk over books/shoe boxes with gaps of 1,5 m at normal pace for 3-5 minutes, increase speed or decrease gaps if the task could be performed easily):

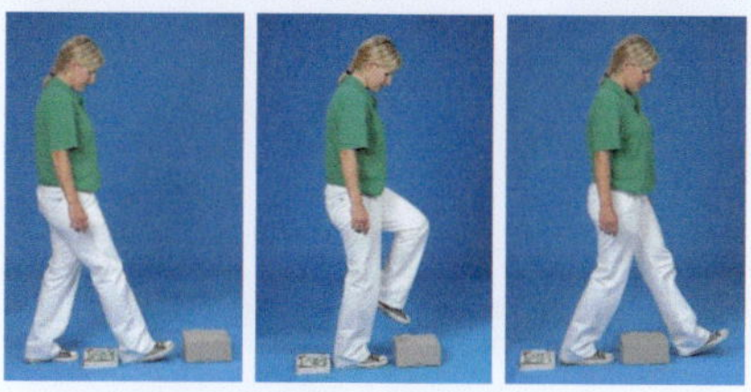

4. Walking round obstacles

(walk round books/shoe boxes with gaps of 1,5 m at normal pace in zigzag pattern for 3-5 minutes, increase speed or decrease gaps if the task could be performed easily):

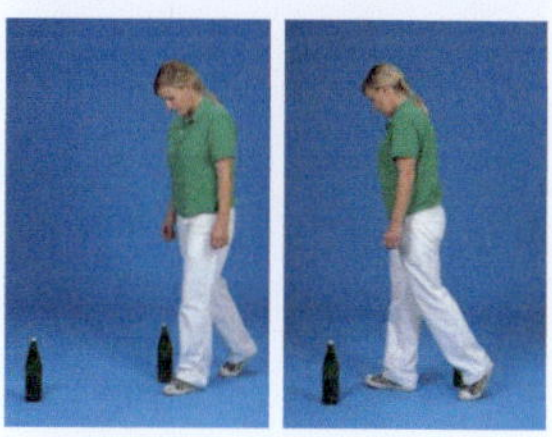

5. Walking slowly

(walk along a line as slowly as possible, repeat for 3-5 min)

Fig. 2.11 Exercises for gait disorders

6. Walking like a stork

(walk along a line while lifting the knees very high, walk slowly if you feel secure and repeat for 3-5 minutes):

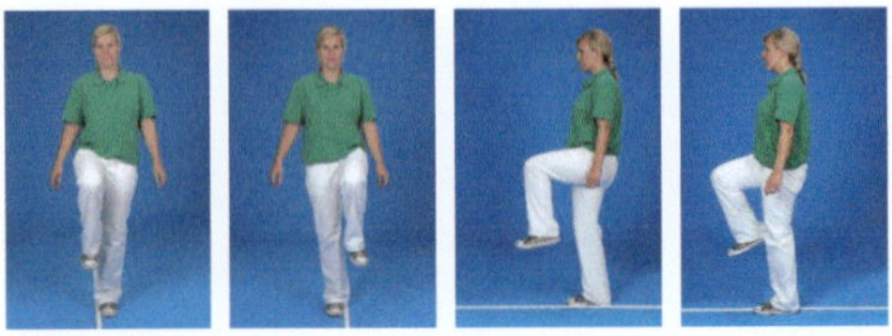

7. Walking and crossing your feet

(cross the feed during walking, increase the difficulty by crossing the arms in front of the chest, repeat for 3-5 minutes):

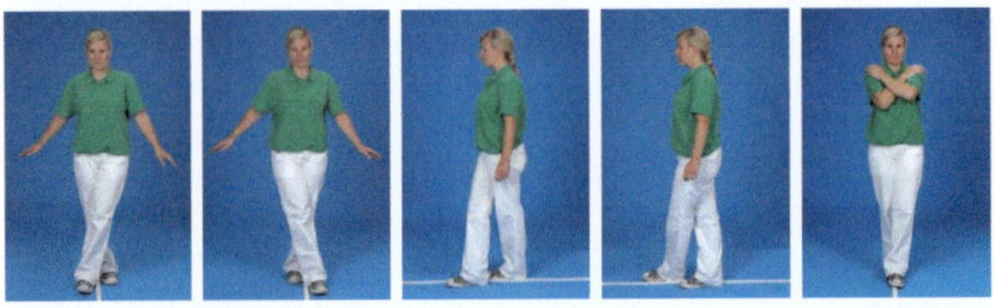

8. Tightrope-walking

(place one foot close to the front of the other during walking, increase difficulty by reducing the gap and by crossing the arms in front of the chest, repeat for 3-5 minutes):

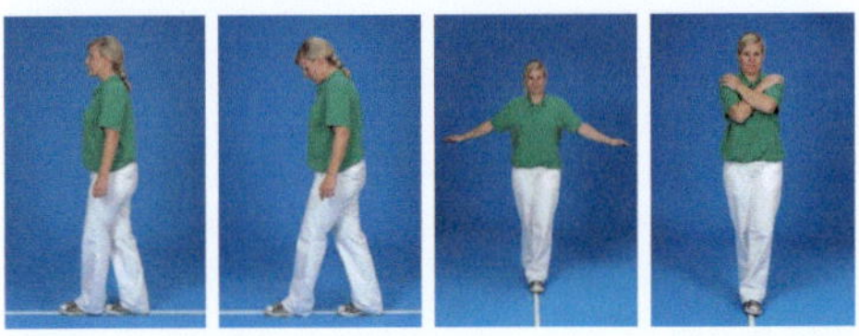

9. Walking over uneven ground

(walk over a thick, folded blanket or a foam mat, perform exercise 5, 6 and 8-13 also on this uneven ground (if possible), use a chair as a security handle (if necessary), repeat for 3-5 minutes):

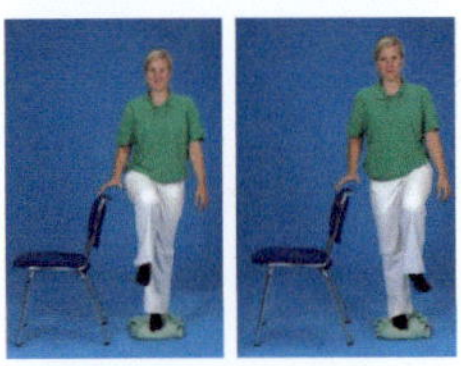

10. Standing on one leg

(standing on one leg as shown below for 15-30 seconds, repeat 10x for each leg):

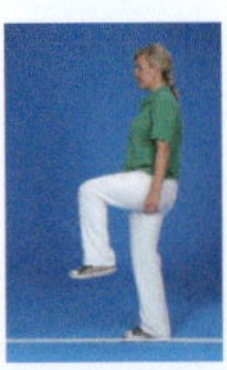

Fig. 2.11 (continued)

11. Alternate the foot on a step

(stand in front of a step (e. g. thick book) and alternate the feet placed on top of the step, perform this 3x 1-2 minutes):

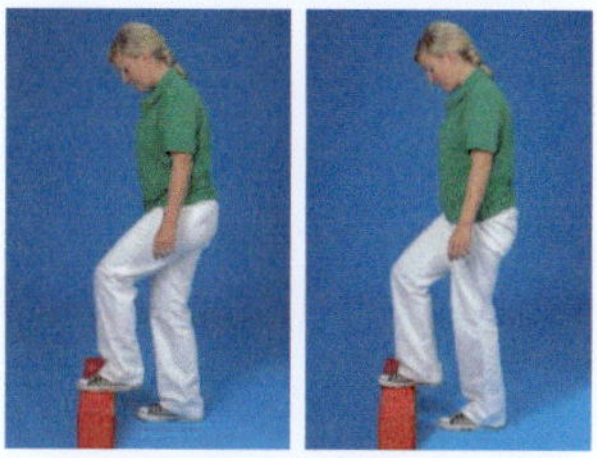

12. Walking on the spot

(walk on the spot and lift your feet higher and higher if possible, increase the time in which you are standing on one leg, perform this 3x 1-2 minutes):

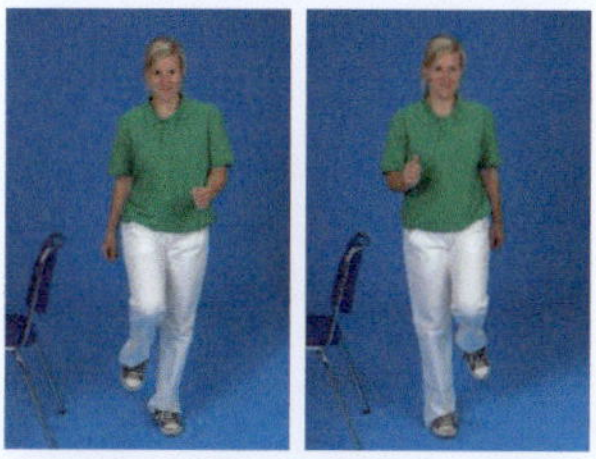

13. Jumping on the spot

(dont't perform this if you suffer from leg pain or after a recent surgery, start to jump from one leg to the other, continue jumping with both legs, increase high if you feel stable, repeat jumping with and without fixation of a frontal target, perform this 3x 1-2 minutes):

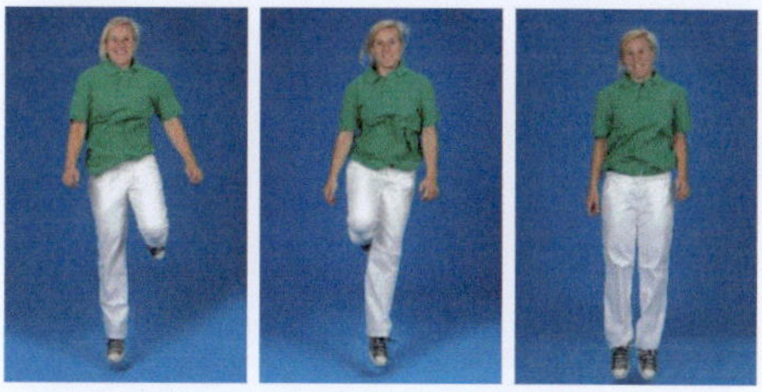

Fig. 2.11 (continued)

The more complex the vestibular disorder (e.g., after head trauma, stroke) and the more additional (cardiovascular) disorders prevail, the more difficult and longer is PT required as part of a neurorehabilitation program with a specialized team. In general, the success of therapy is limited by age, peripheral neuropathy, comorbidities (e.g., cardiovascular disorders, diabetes), (multiple) drug intake, vision deficits, cognitive and/or psychiatric impairment (Klatt et al. 2015).

1. Standing up and sitting down

(sit down on a chair without armrests and stand up repeatedly, perform this 3x for 1-2 minutes with and without fixation of an object at eye level):

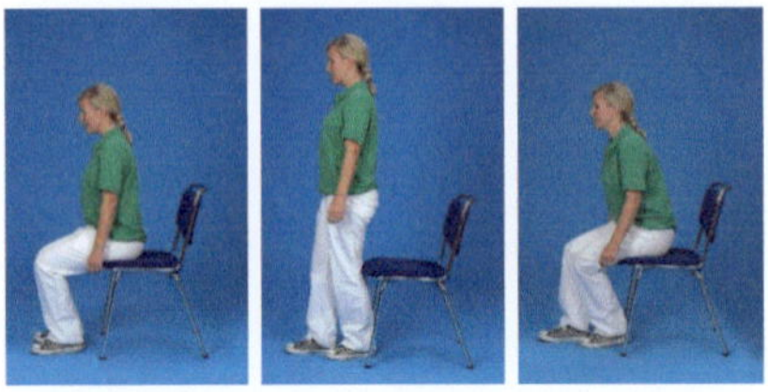

2. Picking up an object diagonally

(Pick an object from the floor on one side and put it to the other side, perform this from a standing or sitting position for 3x 1-2 minutes):

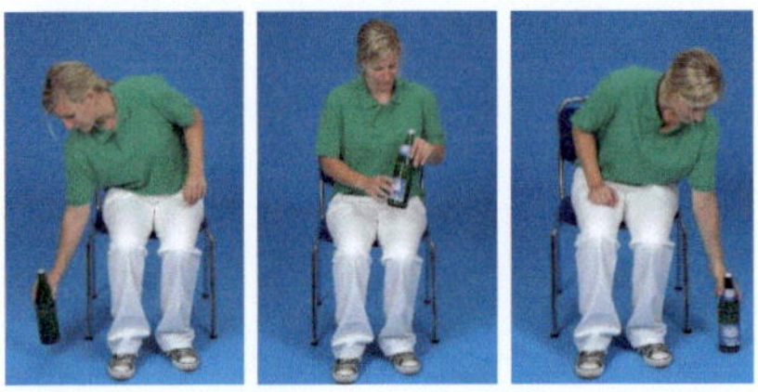

3. Making circling movements with an object while following it visually

(lift an object (e. g. ball) above the head with both hands and make circling movements with it, the eyes should fixate the object, perform this from a standing or sitting position for 3x 1-2 minutes):

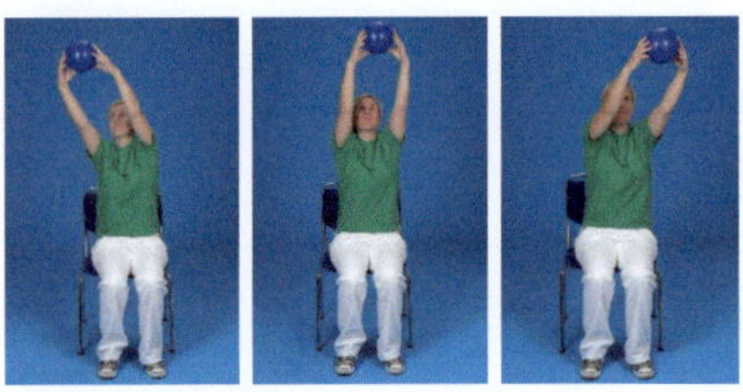

4. Standing on one leg

(standing on one leg as shown below for 15-30 seconds, repeat 10x for each leg):

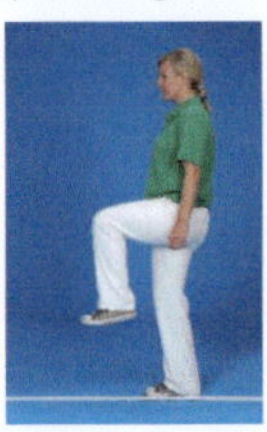

Fig. 2.12 Exercises for balance disorders

5. Tandem stance

(place one foot directly in front of the other (heel and toes touches), change the foot order after every 30 seconds, repeat this 10x):

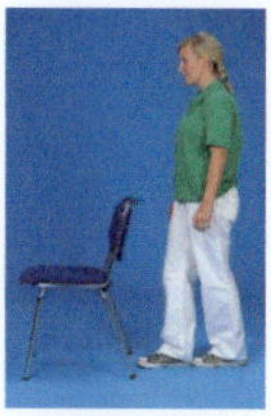

6. Close stance

(place the feet together as close as possible and stand still as possible, repeat this 10x for 30 seconds):

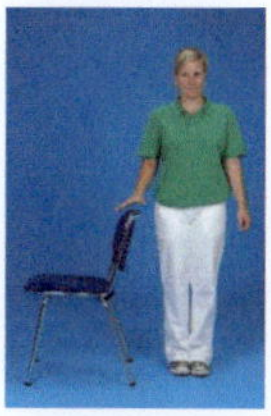

7. Standing on an uneven surface

(stand on a thick, folded blanket or a foam mat and stand still as possible, start with feet hip-width apart and reduce the distance if feel safe, repeat this 10x for 30 seconds):

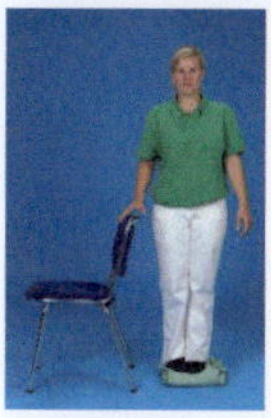

8. Walking on the spot

(walk on the spot and lift your feet higher and higher if possible, increase the time in which you are standing on one leg, perform this 3x 1-2 minutes):

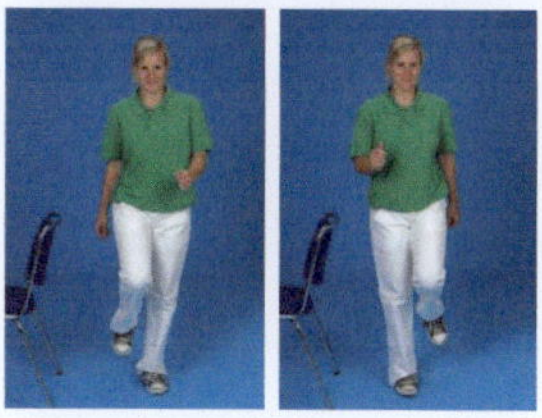

Fig. 2.12 (continued)

9. Throwing a ball while following it visually

(stand with feet hip-width apart and throw a ball from one hand to the other, follow it visually, start at chest hight and elevate the position if you progress):

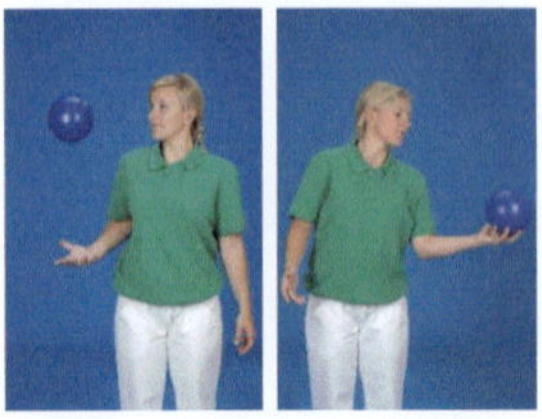

10. Alternate the foot on a step

(stand in front of a step (e. g. thick book) and alternate the feet placed on top of the step, perform this 3x 1-2 minutes):

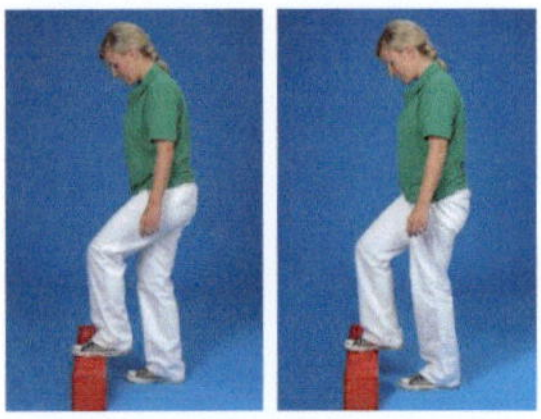

11. Jumping on the spot

(don't perform this if you suffer from leg pain or after a recent surgery, start to jump from one leg to the other, continue jumping with both legs, increase high if you feel stable, repeat jumping with and without fixation of a frontal target, perform this 3x 1-2 minutes):

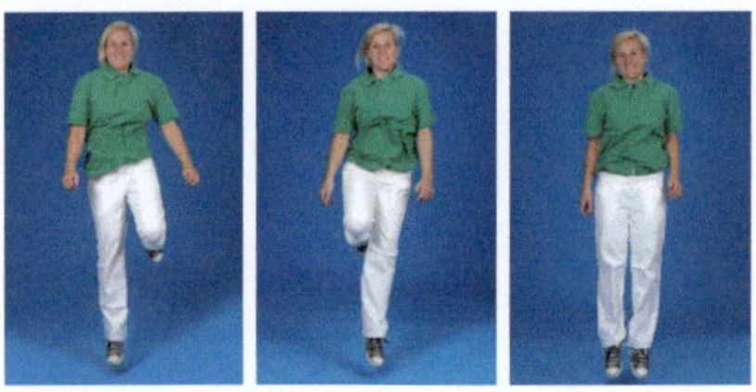

12. Walking slowly

(walk along a line as slowly as possible, repeat for 3-5 min)

13. Stepping over obstacles

(walk over books/shoe boxes with gaps of 1,5 m at normal pace for 3-5 minutes, increase speed or decrease gaps if the task could be performed easily):

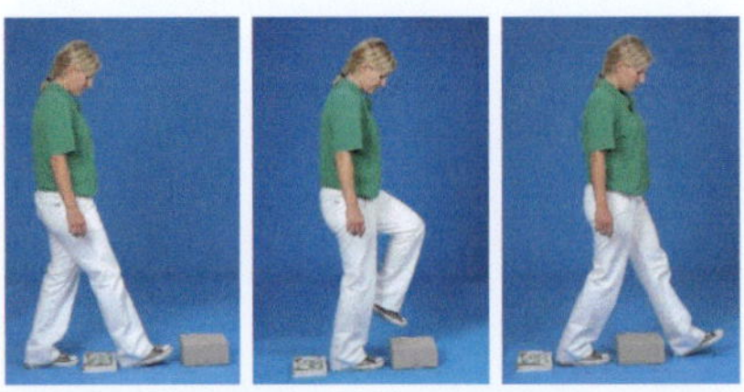

Fig. 2.12 (continued)

14. Walking like a stork

(walk along a line while lifting the knees very high, walk slowly if you feel secure and repeat for 3-5 minutes):

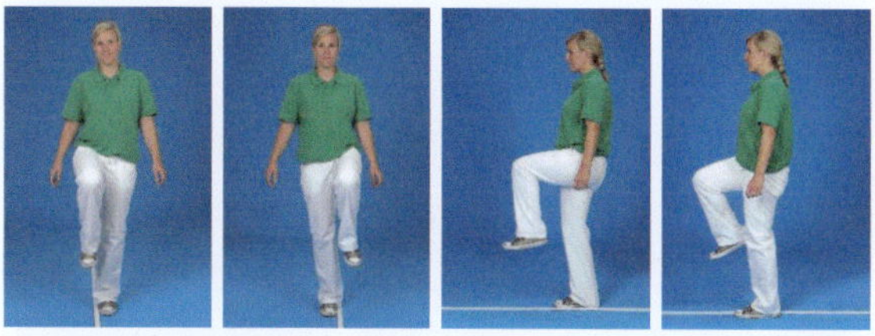

15. Tightrope-walking

(place one foot close to the front of the other during walking, increase difficulty by reducing the gap and by crossing the arms in front of the chest, repeat for 3-5 minutes):

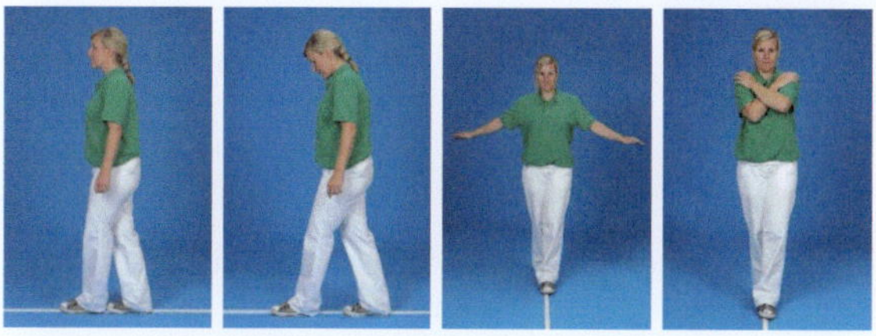

16. Walking over uneven ground

(walk over a thick, folded blanket or a foam mat, perform exercise 12, 14 and 15 also on this uneven ground (if possible), use a chair as a security handle (if necessary), repeat for 3-5 minutes):

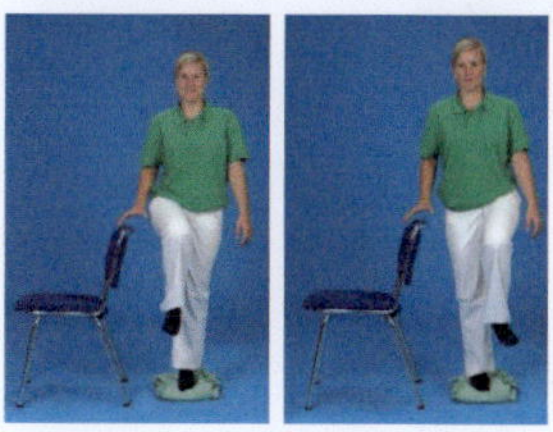

Fig. 2.12 (continued)

2.3.3 Rehabilitation Technology in Vestibular Disorders

2.3.3.1 Background

Within the last decade, technical innovation initiated a fundamental change in vestibular rehabilitation. This is due to the increased number of vestibular patients in clinics and practices and to the enhanced efficacy of specific devices for the treatment of numerous vestibular diseases. The solutions range from large and expensive devices for clinical use in hospitals to smart tools for home application. Beside the simple guidance through rehabilitation exercises, active devices can improve and speed-up the rehabilitation. Such active devices mainly provide feedback about the

1. Horizontal saccades

(look alternating on your index fingers which are hold vertically in front 30 cm apart, continue for 3x 1 min):

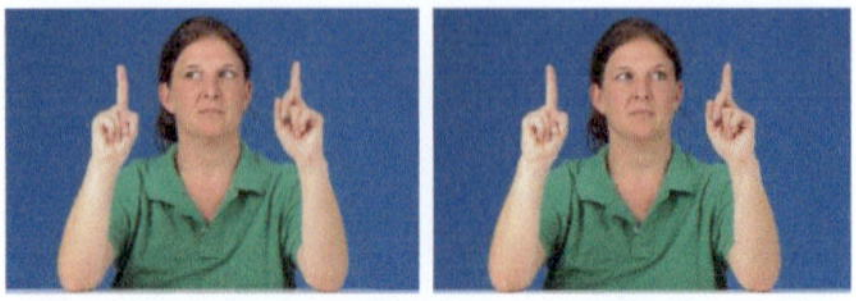

2. Vertical saccades

(look alternating on your index fingers which are hold horizontally in front 30 cm apart, continue for 3x 1 min):

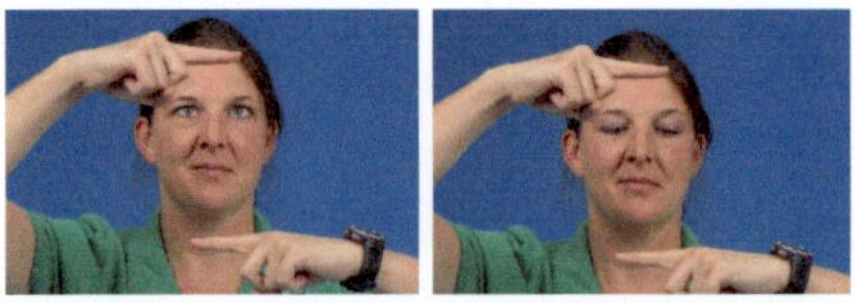

3. Horizontal smooth pursuit

(fixate with your eyes (not moving the head) your slowly horizontal moving thumb, continue for 3x 1 minute):

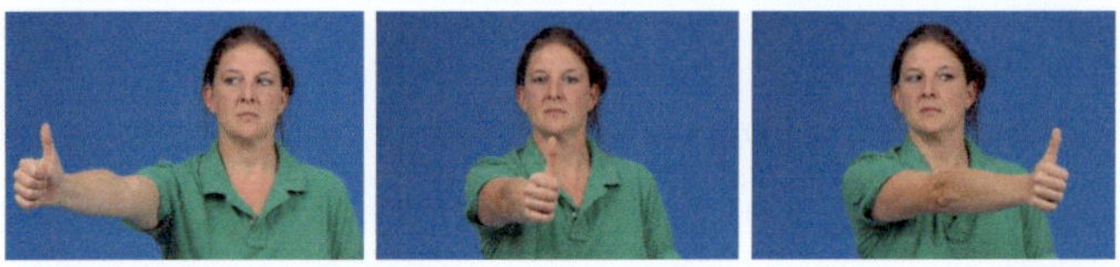

4. Vertical smooth pursuit

(fixate with your eyes (not moving the head) your slowly vertical moving thumb, continue for 3x 1 minute):

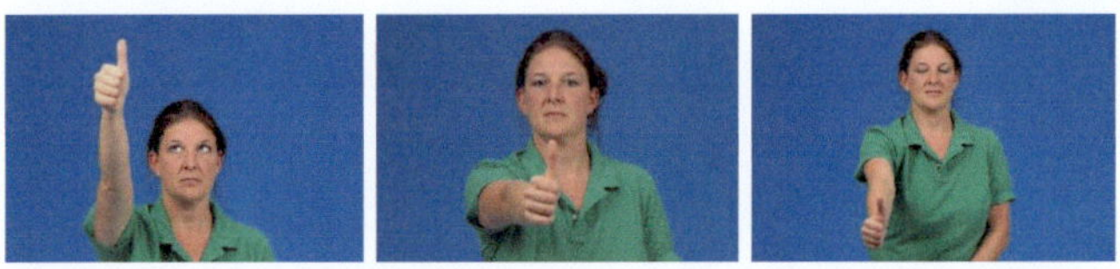

5. Turning the head with gaze fixation

(fixate your thumb in front while turning the head from one side to the other, continue for 3x 1 minute):

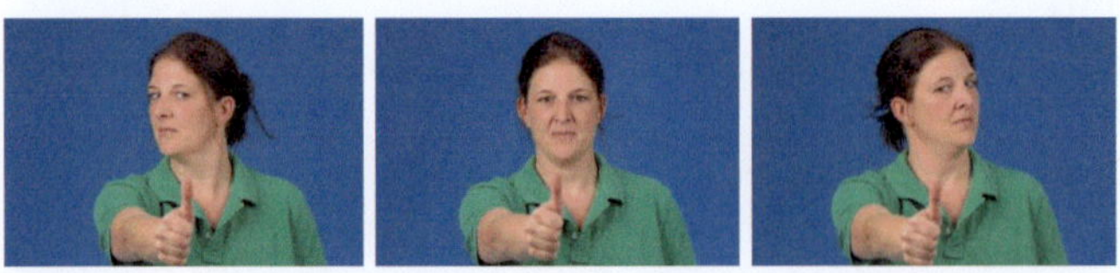

Fig. 2.13 Exercises for acute vertigo/dizziness

6. Nodding with gaze fixation

(fixate your thumb in front while move the head up and down, continue for 3x 1 minute):

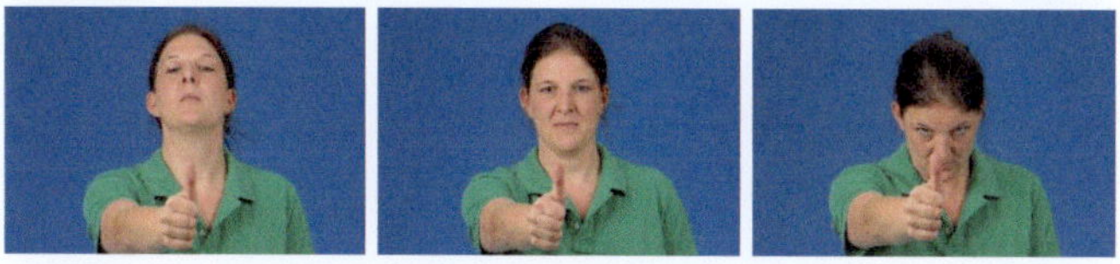

7. Lateral inclination with gaze fixation

(fixate your thumb in front while tilting the head from one side to the other, continue for 3x 1 minute):

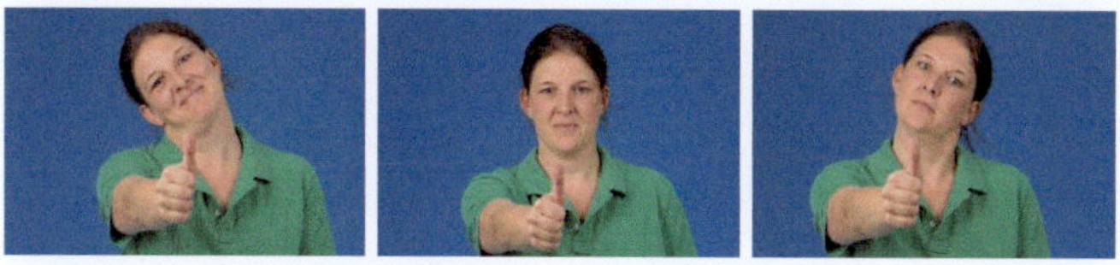

8. Upper body and head rotation

(fixate your thumbs which are upright in your clasped hands in front while turning the upper body from one side to the other, continue for 3x 1 minute):

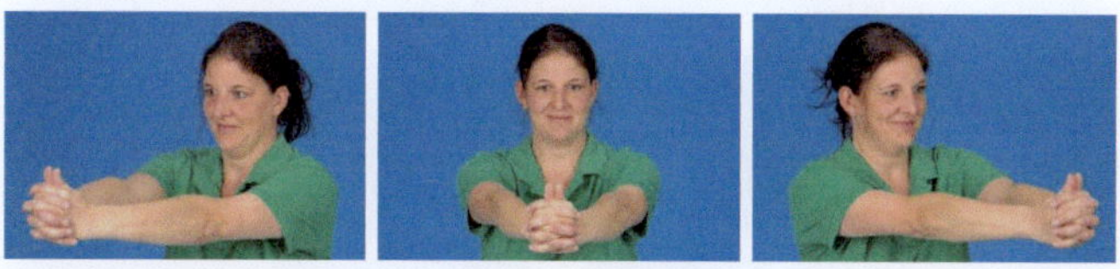

9. Standing up and sitting down

(sit down on a chair without armrests and stand up repeatedly, perform this 3x for 1-2 minutes with and without fixation of an object at eye level):

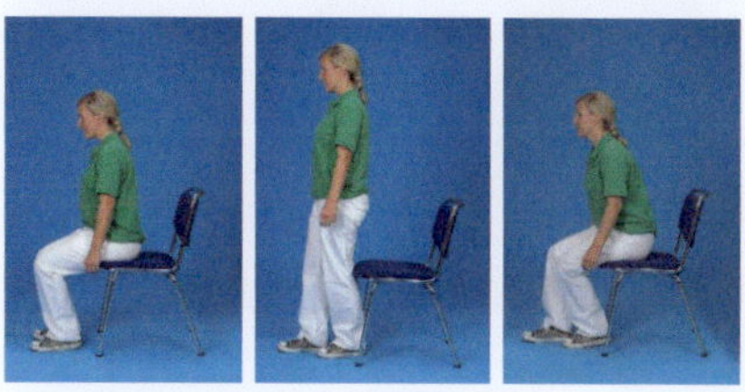

10. Picking up an object diagonally

(Pick an object from the floor on one side and put it to the other side, perform this from a standing or sitting position for 3x 1-2 minutes):

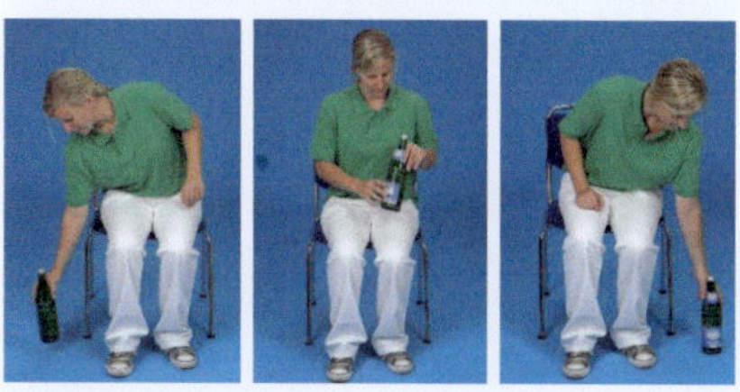

Fig. 2.13 (continued)

11. Standing on one leg

(standing on one leg as shown below for 15-30 seconds, repeat 10x for each leg):

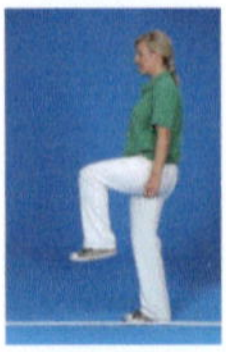

12. Standing on an uneven surface

(stand on a thick, folded blanket or a foam mat and stand still as possible, start with feet hip-width apart and reduce the distance if feel safe, repeat this 10x for 30 seconds):

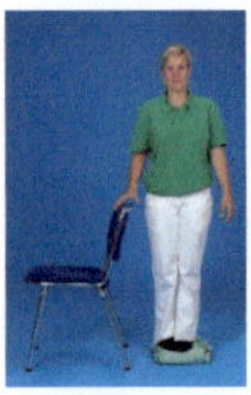

13. Tightrope-walking

(place one foot close to the front of the other during walking, increase difficulty by reducing the gap and by crossing the arms in front of the chest, repeat for 3-5 minutes):

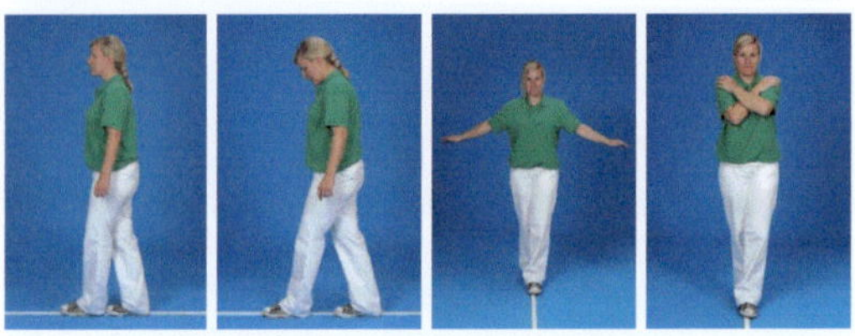

14. Stepping over obstacles

(walk over books/shoe boxes with gaps of 1,5 m at normal pace for 3-5 minutes, increase speed or decrease gaps if the task could be performed easily):

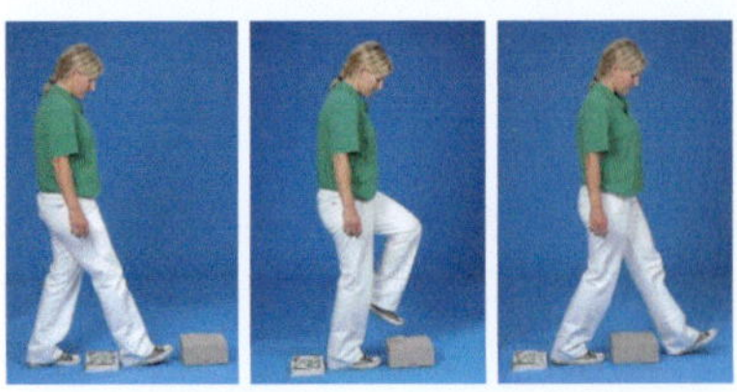

15. Walking while moving the head

(walk 3-5 minutes with and without a target fixation, change head position every three steps):

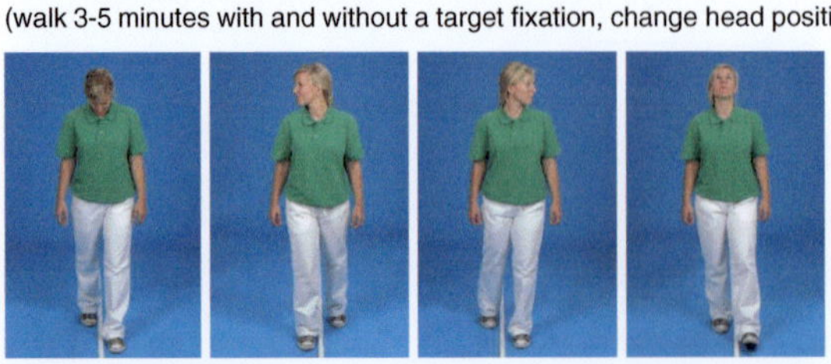

Fig. 2.13 (continued)

current sway to the patient. The feedback signalizes the specific lack of postural control while the task is performed. Thus, the patient can correct the posture and memorize unconsciously the safe (normal) range of body sway. Such a technology is particularly very helpful in patients which require a long-lasting conventional vestibular rehabilitation or if other rehabilitation approaches were not successful (e.g., in otolith disorders, bilateral vestibulopathy, presbyvestibulopathy). Especially the latter group of patients benefit from a more effective vestibular rehabilitation with feedback devices since only short exercises (typically 20 s for each) are required for a couple of consecutive days. Thus, elderly patients don't have to perform exhausting tasks for weeks to benefit from a rehabilitation program. The same holds true for patients which suffer from severe dizziness or vertigo.

> Nowadays, vestibular rehabilitation relies more and more on technical devices. Especially active devices which provide feedback in relation to the patient's postural control could increase the rehabilitation efficacy.

2.3.3.2 Smartphone Applications

Currently, approximately 3.8 million apps are available for iOS-based device smartphones, and 2.8 million for Android-based devices. It could be assumed that a small share of these apps has the potential to facilitate healthcare for both patients and clinicians. Research has demonstrated the use of healthcare apps in decision-making, symptom tracking, and exercise assistance. There is a lack, however, of systematic evaluation of the quality of vertigo apps. Third-party health app libraries, such as ORCHA app finder, provide quality assessments of health apps, but up to now they did not include vertigo apps. Many apps are freely or at low cost available to patients, and it is imperative that clinicians are aware of their benefits and limitations, to establish whether they can be integrated into clinical use.

It could be helpful if the app quality was already assessed using the validated 23-item Mobile App Rating Scale (MARS). This tool has been demonstrated to judge at least the basic functionality. It assesses app engagement, functionality, aesthetics, information, subjective quality, and app-specific impact. Scores are rated on a 5-point scale (1 = inadequate, 5 = excellent).

There are already a few apps available for symptom tracking and some to provide exercise guidance. Some apps stated to be developed by healthcare professionals for symptom tracking (e.g., Meniere's monitor, DizzyCAM®, DizzyTrack®) and some give advice for rehabilitation exercises (e.g., Healing vertigo, BPPV relief, VOR neuro balance, BPPV treatment, Positional vertigo app, Tebonin® app). The participation of related healthcare professionals could also signalize a more serious application. Until now, the efficacy was not investigated in controlled studies for any vertigo app in the app-stores. Some new developments are not distributed over app-stores (e.g., VestAid® = individualized and controlled VOR-training, Hovareshti et al. 2021). An alternative distribution (e.g., hardware connected) could bypass the app-stores. Because of the opportunities of the technology and the growing acceptance of technical tools for home use, this area seems to develop rapidly within the next years. However, it will be always an issue to assess the quality before the use of a vestibular rehabilitation app.

Smartphone apps are already available for symptom tracking and rehabilitation exercise guidance. However, it is a very small but growing market. Quality assessment is very important before an app should be used. Unfortunately, no RCTs were performed until now to show the efficacy of any treatment app.

2.3.3.3 Feedback Devices

Even if, in the sum of all training approaches, balance training is assessed as effective with high evidence, there are very large differences between the training approaches in terms of therapeutic success (McDonnell and Hillier 2015). Patients with multimodal dizziness in elderly age are particularly difficult to treat with conventional balance training. A meta-study was able to determine only minor effects of this therapy approach in the group of elderly patients and these only in a proportion of the participants (Crocker et al. 2013). Also, despite increased prevention measures, the risk of falls in elderly patients cannot be significantly reduced (Choi and Hector 2012). Machine-aided approaches, especially with intuitive feedback signals, seem to be much more effective and successful here. The same applies to other patient groups. These aspects should be considered when selecting the appropriate therapy for vestibular rehabilitation. The feedback systems described below can be used depending on the type and severity of the vestibular disorder and the resulting risk of falling as well as the individual suitability of the patient. Particularly, effective approaches are to be preferred in any case in the case of a high risk of falls, chronification because of previous treatment failure, or low physical resilience of the patient.

A program that is specifically tailored to the individual deficits of the respective patient can be viewed as the ideal concept for feedback training. In addition, the feedback signal should not disturb or influence the perception of environmental stimuli. In addition, feedback information should not lead to sensory conflict situations, especially if they contain parts of a virtual reality (e.g., depiction of movements in space).

The general functional principle of feedback training is based on an unconscious learning process. During the training, the patient learns to use information about body conditions such as tendon tension, joint position, visual and proprioceptive stimulus patterns to a greater extent in the context of balance control. The feedback signal helps the body during training to modulate the individual normal range of these parameters for the corresponding sensorimotor condition. A reassessment of vegetative afferents takes place. If this goal is achieved, it is possible for the patient to maintain an approximately normal body stability even without the feedback signal.

2.3.3.4 Auditory Feedback

An auditory feedback training could be applied in patients with a sufficient bilateral hearing ability. Patients should localize a sound source during performing stance or gait tasks which is activated if the body sway exceeds a pre-set threshold in the specific direction. One device (SwayStar®), which could be also used in gait tasks, contains two angular velocity sensors mounted on an elastic belt, which is positioned on the patient's lower trunk (Fig. 2.14). The transducers are oriented in roll and pitch planes. A software program records and analzes the velocity and angle of trunk movements and calculates the related auditory feedback. Auditory biofeedback is delivered via four loudspeakers placed left, right, in front and back of the patient (5 m × 4 m test environment). The loudness of the acoustic signal is increased linearly with increasing angular velocity from 60 to 95 dB SPL. Studies have shown an effective training for nearly 50% of all participating patients (Basta et al. 2008). One aspect which could negatively influence the outcome (beside impaired bilateral or unilateral hearing) is that the patient must learn how to react if a tone from a specific direction occurs. Patients which can learn the procedure show a significant reduction of sway after the first week of daily training. Another approach is the use of headphones which provide acoustic feedback both lateral directions and simulating the anterior/posterior direction (e.g., Equivert®). The sway measurement is realized by accelerometers in the headphones which allows only the performance of stance tasks. The sway measurement on the head is an additional limitation of the method since the center of gravity (located in the pelvic center) is the regulated parameter during maintaining postural control. No controlled studies have shown the efficacy of such a headphone-based system so far. More promising is the auditory feedback provided via headphones during stance tasks by the THERA-Trainer "coro"® since the sway is measured continuously on the hip (Fuchs et al. 2020). Results from the application in patients should be available soon.

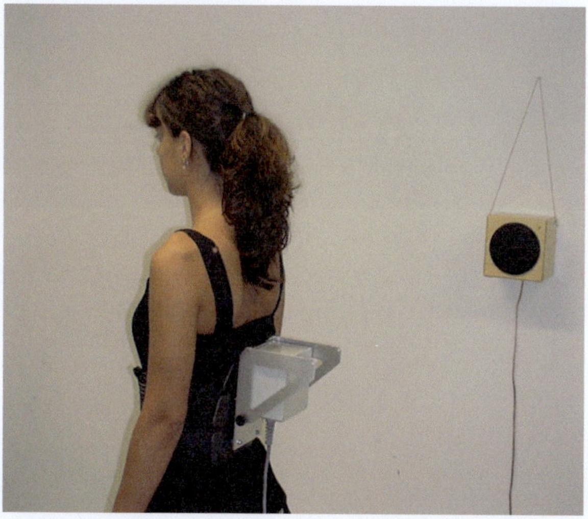

Fig. 2.14 Example of an auditory feedback device application (SwayStar®)

Studies showed recently that the auditory input itself could influence postural control in a negative and positive fashion (Anton et al., 2019). The specific effect depends on the task, the auditory signal, and the age of the patient (Basta et al. 2023). Especially gait tasks are more frequently affected by an auditory stimulation. It is questionable if this holds also true for the directed auditory feedback signal applied in the feedback systems but it is a possible additional limitation of the auditory feedback training.

2.3.3.5 Visual Feedback

Sensory neurofeedback for the treatment of balance disorders was first used using a visual feedback signal during exercises on a force platform. In this approach, the estimation of the center of gravity by measuring the center of pressure within the foot surfaces is not used to assess balance performance. Rather, the patient is informed visually about the position of the center of pressure. This offers the opportunity to use this additional information as a feedback signal in the regulation of balance and to apply it in training programs. It is often offered to control the position of the visualized center of pressure to certain end points (e.g., Balance Master®) or for gaming tasks in a virtual visual environment (Balance Quest Prime®, Fig. 2.15). It is important that the plates are force transducer devices that calculate the pressure point and not the acceleration of the entire plate. In the latter case,

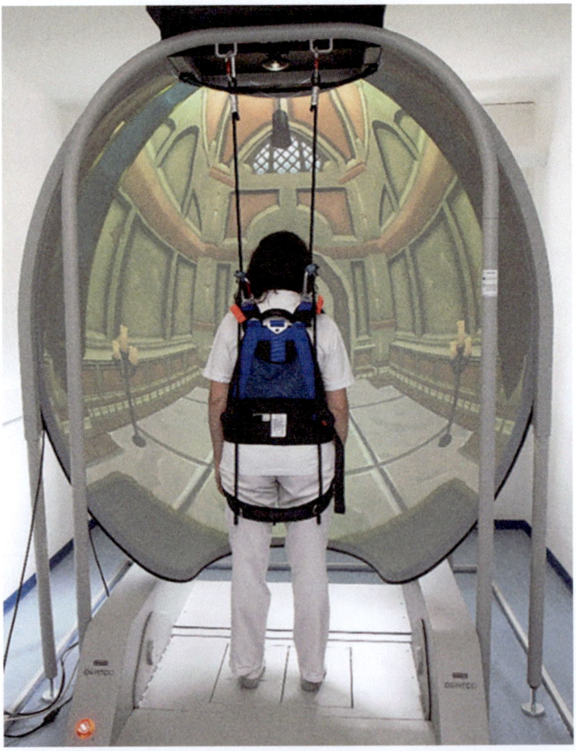

Fig. 2.15 Example of a visual feedback device (Balance Quest®)

non-physiological movements would be necessary for control, which hardly support central compensation. Force plates coupled with visual feedback may be superior to conventional balance training (McDonnell and Hillier 2015). The use of a virtual, visual reality is generally not recommended, as movements are often shown (e.g., jumping, skiing) that trigger sensory conflicts due to the patient's actual standing situation. However, the balance training with visual feedback on a force plate can enhance the stance stability in specific patient groups such as unilateral vestibular loss (Rossi-Izquierdo et al. 2011), Parkinson's disease (Rossi-Izquierdo et al. 2013), or presbyvestibulopathy (Soto-Varela et al. 2021) even if the effectiveness of other techniques was shown to be superior in these studies.

Because of recent developments, it is important to note that balance systems developed as toys should also be regarded as such. In addition to the lack of approval for medical use, the large market advantage in the toy segment (realistic virtual, visual reality) and the challenging nature of the tasks are a hindrance in the treatment of patients with severe balance disorders. Moderate improvements (compared to no treatment) were reported for patients with mild symptoms (Sparrer et al. 2013).

The fundamental disadvantage of systems with force transducer plates is that they can only be used for standing exercises and that the determination of the shift in the body's center of gravity is indirect. Since the feedback cannot be followed exactly by shifting the center of foot pressure, feedback training based on this signal is not optimally adapted to the patient's body swaying. The effectiveness of the training is therefore limited from the outset.

2.3.3.6 Galvanic Feedback

Galvanic feedback was used by a device some years ago, and it is not clear if it will come back to the market in this fashion. However, the idea is interesting, and it is likely that this was not the last approach in this field. The device (BrainPort®) consists of a controller and tethered Intra-Oral Device (IOD). The IOD and tether include a circuit with 100 electrodes (10 × 10 array), and a Micro-Electro-Mechanical Systems (MEMS) accelerometer for sensing head tilt and motion. The oral unit also contains circuitry to convert the controller signals into individualized zero to +18 Volt monophasic pulsed stimuli on the 100-point distributed ground tongue display which are applied as a permanent feedback signal in relation to head movements during stance tasks. The feedback signal is centered at the beginning of each training task during a stable head position. All deviations from this head position led to a change of stimulation side within the electrode array in relation to the head movement (Danilov et al., 2006). In theory, the specific galvanic input via the trigeminal nerve should enhance the efficacy of the vestibular rehabilitation training (e.g., standing for 20 min on foam or with eyes closed). The training is exhausting and unfortunately not effective if compared to a placebo application in most of the patient groups. However, the concept of a translingual neural stimulation to provide an arousal for vestibular rehabilitation is still promising. A device which delivers continuous electrical stimulation on the tongue during the performance of vestibular rehabilitation tasks (PoNS®, Fig. 2.16) has proven to improve the rehabilitation

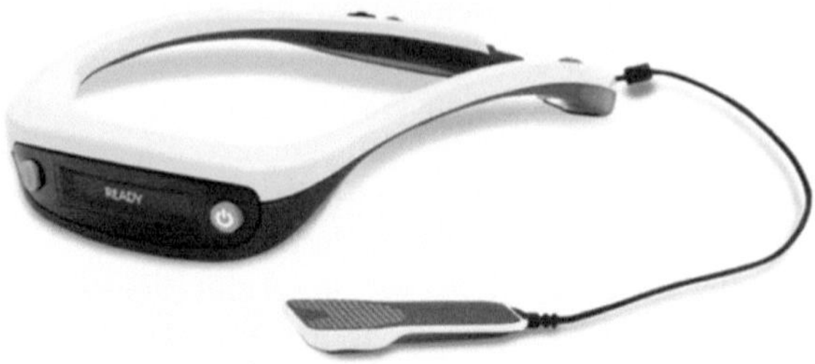

Fig. 2.16 Example of a galvanic feedback device (PoNS®)

benefit of physical therapy in patients with multiple sclerosis or moderate traumatic brain injury (Hou et al. 2022).

An emerging technique is the continuous application of a noisy electrical (galvanic) stimulation (nGVS) on the mastoid bilaterally (e.g., Soterix medical®, NeuroConn®). The application of subliminal stochastic signals can in general improve the detectability and thereby perception of biological signals (Wuehr et al. 2023a). Blurry pictures, e.g., are better visible with the right amount of noise added to the weak signal. For the vestibular system, subtle currents can improve postural balance and gait in patients with bilateral vestibular loss. There is some evidence that there is a moderate effect of a more effective rehabilitation by nGVS in patients with a bilateral vestibular loss (McLaren et al. 2022; Wuehr et al. 2023b).

2.3.3.7 Vibrotactile Feedback

The approach of vibrotactile neurofeedback training is to ensure normal posture or balance even with reduced vestibular, visual, or proprioceptive input by conveying the missing information through tactile stimulation. The vibrotactile sense is particularly well suited to this, as it is processed intuitively and leads to an involuntary correction of posture. Furthermore, the vibrotactile stimulus, in contrast to the visual or acoustic stimulus, does not impede the acquisition of information from the environment.

There are two different approaches in general. One with a permanent vibration signal depending on the body sway and a second with a signal-like stimulation only when specific swaying ranges are exceeded. The first variant is implemented, for example, by a system (BalanceBelt®) that is recommended for permanent wear. Unfortunately, the expected prolonged activation of the numerous vibration stimulators in this system can lead to habituation of the vibration receptors in the skin. The system is worn on the hip, where the angular velocity is also measured. However, placebo-controlled studies which investigate the effectiveness of this approach are still pending. A recent study showed a subjective increase of stability in pre-selected patients with a severe bilateral vestibular loss (Kingma et al. 2019). The pre-selection was based on the patient's judgment after 2 h of continuous application. In addition, a long-term training effect is unlikely (Ballardini et al. 2020).

Another system (VibroTactile®) uses signal stimulation only if specific fluctuation values are exceeded. These thresholds are specific to each direction of body sway and should be set by a therapist. The vibratory stimulation is applied on the waist. This system is only applicable during stance tasks on a force platform. The sway is calculated based on pressure measurements on the sole of the foot. Thus, all limitations apply for this method as described for the platform training above (see visual feedback). There are no published clinical trials available now on the efficacy of the device. However, a recent study showed very limited effects on stance stability after the training with a similar concepted experimental device (Kodama et al. 2019).

The single device with vibratory feedback which could be used for vestibular rehabilitation in stance and gait tasks is currently the Vertiguard®-system (mobile posturography). The feedback thresholds are set by the system itself based on the patient's age and sex and the specific sensorimotor training condition.

Before the actual training, the patient completes a body sway analysis in everyday situations, with the body swaying being continuously measured close to the body's center of gravity. The results are compared with internally stored, age and sex-related standard values. This makes it possible to objectively identify and quantify the individual deficits in terms of the patient's postural control. In the subsequent training, the patient should reduce the body sway in the conditions that are problematic with the help of the additional vibrotactile signal and thus improve the body balance in everyday life.

The training system consists of a control device that is worn on a hip belt and continuously measures body swaying at the body's center of gravity, as well as four vibration stimulators attached to the same belt at 90° offset (Fig. 2.17).

During the individualized vibrotactile neurofeedback training, the selected tasks are repeated five times on a maximum of 10 training days. As with the body sway analysis, each condition is only completed for a maximum of 20 s during training. The extremely short exercise duration of max 20 s reduces the physical strain of the training. This proves to be a great advantage, especially for elderly patients.

Vibration is well suited as a feedback signal since it is processed intuitively and do not impair other inputs of the vestibular system (e.g., vision, hearing). The vibratory feedback could be applied permanently depending on body sway or as a signal-like stimulation only when specific swaying ranges are exceeded. The latter mode has a proven long-term effect. An individualized vestibular training is most effective.

The effectiveness of individualized vibrotactile neurofeedback training (iNFT) in everyday sensorimotor conditions has been reported in patients with vestibular disorders of various origins in double-blind placebo-controlled studies. In patients with multifactorial dizziness in old age, uncompensated unilateral and bilateral vestibulopathies and in Parkinson's patients, a significant reduction in body swaying and the risk of falls has been demonstrated (Basta et al. 2011; Rossi-Izquierdo et al. 2013; Brugnera et al. 2015; Soto-Varela et al. 2021).

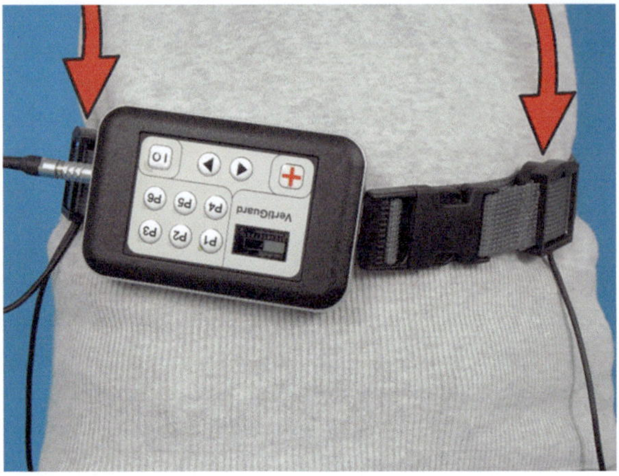

Fig. 2.17 Example of a vibrotactile feedback device application (Vertiguard®). The arrows indicate vibratory stimulators which are activated by the main unit. The main unit is connected "head-down" on the same belt for a better usability by the patient

However, the results depend on the severity and combination of the vestibular disorders. Limited success has been reported for this method after removal of an acoustic neuroma, in Menière's disease or in patients with a neurovascular conflict.

Patients who use the benefit of mobility after the training in everyday life shows a long-lasting or permanent effect. The central compensation or habituation is maintained and further strengthened by the regained motor activity. In the case of progressive diseases (e.g., in Parkinson's disease), however, the therapeutic effect is overlaid again for a short time. The interval for repeat training is then between 3 and 6 months. Nevertheless, long-term success is always very individual and should be checked regularly (e.g., every 6–12 months in elderly patients) using a body sway analysis.

References

Anton K, Ernst A, Basta D (2019) Auditory influence on postural control during stance tasks in different acoustic conditions. J Vestib Res 29(6):287–294. https://doi.org/10.3233/VES-190674

Ballardini G, Florio V, Canessa A et al (2020) Vibrotactile feedback for improving standing balance. Front Bioeng Biotechnol 8:94. https://doi.org/10.3389/fbioe.2020.00094

Basta D, Singbartl F, Todt I et al (2008) Vestibular rehabilitation by auditory feedback in otolith disorders. Gait Posture 28(3):397–404. https://doi.org/10.1016/j.gaitpost.2008.01.006

Basta D, Rossi-Izquierdo M, Soto-Varela A et al (2011) Efficacy of a vibrotactile neurofeedback training in stance and gait conditions for the treatment of balance deficits: a double-blind, placebo-controlled multicenter study. Otol Neurotol 32(9):1492–1499. https://doi.org/10.1097/MAO.0b013e31823827ec

Basta D, Borsellino L, Anton K et al (2023) Influence of auditory information on postural control during different gait tasks in the elderly. J Int Adv Otol 19(1):22–27. https://doi.org/10.5152/iao.2023.22671

Berg K, Norman KE (1996) Functional assessment of balance and gait. Clin Geriatr Med 12(4):705–723

Brown KE, Whitney SL, Marchetti GF et al (2006) Physical therapy for central vestibular dysfunction. Arch Phys Med Rehabil 87(1):76–81. https://doi.org/10.1016/j.apmr.2005.08.003

Brugnera C, Bittar RS, Greters ME et al (2015) Effects of vibrotactile vestibular substitution on vestibular rehabilitation—preliminary study. Braz J Otorhinolaryngol 81(6):616–621. https://doi.org/10.1016/j.bjorl.2015.08.013

Choi M, Hector M (2012) Effectiveness of intervention programs in preventing falls: a systematic review of recent 10 years and meta-analysis. J Am Med Dir Assoc 13(2):188 e113–188 e121. https://doi.org/10.1016/j.jamda.2011.04.022

Crocker T, Young J, Forster A et al (2013) The effect of physical rehabilitation on activities of daily living in older residents of long-term care facilities: systematic review with meta-analysis. Age Ageing 42(6):682–688. https://doi.org/10.1093/ageing/aft133

Danilov YP, Tyler ME, Skinner KL et al. (2006) Efficacy of electrotactile vestibular substitution in patients with bilateral vestibular and central balance loss. Conf Proc IEEE Eng Med Biol Soc Suppl:6605–6609. doi:https://doi.org/10.1109/IEMBS.2006.260899

Dieterich M, Brandt T (1999) Episodic vertigo related to migraine (90 cases): vestibular migraine? J Neurol 246(10):883–892

Ekvall Hansson E, Mansson NO, Ringsberg KA et al (2006) Dizziness among patients with whiplash-associated disorder: a randomized controlled trial. J Rehabil Med 38(6):387–390. https://doi.org/10.1080/16501970600768992

Feil K, Bottcher N, Kremmyda O et al (2018) Pharmacotherapy of vestibular disorders, nystagmus and cerebellar disorders. Laryngorhinootologie 97(1):14–23. https://doi.org/10.1055/s-0043-123487

Feller L, Feller G, Ballyram T et al (2020) Interrelations between pain, stress and executive functioning. Br J Pain 14(3):188–194. https://doi.org/10.1177/2049463719889380

Fuchs DK, Egger M, Friedrich P (2020) Audio feedback for device-supported balance training: parameter mapping and influencing factors. Acoustics 2:650–665. https://doi.org/10.3390/acoustics2030034

Hall CD, Herdman SJ, Whitney SL et al (2016) Treatment for vestibular disorders: how does your physical therapist treat dizziness related to vestibular problems? J Neurol Phys Ther 40(2):156. https://doi.org/10.1097/01.NPT.0000481898.55592.6e

Hall CD, Herdman SJ, Whitney SL et al (2022) Vestibular rehabilitation for peripheral vestibular hypofunction: an updated clinical practice guideline from the academy of neurologic physical therapy of the American Physical Therapy Association. J Neurol Phys Ther 46(2):118–177. https://doi.org/10.1097/NPT.0000000000000382

Hansson EE, Persson L, Malmstrom EM (2013) Influence of vestibular rehabilitation on neck pain and cervical range of motion among patients with whiplash-associated disorder: a randomized controlled trial. J Rehabil Med 45(9):906–910. https://doi.org/10.2340/16501977-1197

Hidalgo B, Hall T, Bossert J et al (2017) The efficacy of manual therapy and exercise for treating non-specific neck pain: a systematic review. J Back Musculoskelet Rehabil 30(6):1149–1169. https://doi.org/10.3233/BMR-169615

Hou J, Mohanty R, Chu D et al (2022) Translingual neural stimulation affects resting-state functional connectivity in mild-moderate traumatic brain injury. J Neuroimaging 32(6):1193–1200. https://doi.org/10.1111/jon.13029

Hovareshti P, Roeder S, Holt LS et al (2021) VestAid: a tablet-based technology for objective exercise monitoring in vestibular rehabilitation. Sensors (Basel) 21(24). https://doi.org/10.3390/s21248388

Jahn K (2016) Vertigo and dizziness in children. Handb Clin Neurol 137:353–363. https://doi.org/10.1016/B978-0-444-63437-5.00025-X

Jahn K, Kressig RW, Bridenbaugh SA et al (2015) Dizziness and unstable gait in old age: etiology, diagnosis and treatment. Deutsches Arzteblatt Int 112(23):387–393. https://doi.org/10.3238/arztebl.2015.0387

Kim JS, Newman-Toker DE, Kerber KA et al (2022) Vascular vertigo and dizziness: diagnostic criteria. J Vestib Res 32(3):205–222. https://doi.org/10.3233/VES-210169

Kingma H, Felipe L, Gerards MC et al (2019) Vibrotactile feedback improves balance and mobility in patients with severe bilateral vestibular loss. J Neurol 266(Suppl 1):19–26. https://doi.org/10.1007/s00415-018-9133-z

Klatt BN, Carender WJ, Lin CC et al (2015) A conceptual framework for the progression of balance exercises in persons with balance and vestibular disorders. Phys Med Rehabil Int 2(4)

Kodama K, Yasuda K, Kuznetsov NA et al (2019) Balance training with a vibrotactile biofeedback system affects the dynamical structure of the center of pressure trajectories in chronic stroke patients. Front Hum Neurosci 13:84. https://doi.org/10.3389/fnhum.2019.00084

Langevin P, Fait P, Fremont P et al (2019) Cervicovestibular rehabilitation in adult with mild traumatic brain injury: a randomised controlled trial protocol. BMC Sports Sci Med Rehabil 11:25. https://doi.org/10.1186/s13102-019-0139-3

Leigh RJ, Zee DS (2006) The neurology of eye movements, 4th edn. Oxford University Press, New York

Lemos J, Manto M (2022) Pharmacotherapy of cerebellar and vestibular disorders. Curr Opin Neurol 35(1):118–125. https://doi.org/10.1097/WCO.0000000000001015

McDonnell MN, Hillier SL (2015) Vestibular rehabilitation for unilateral peripheral vestibular dysfunction. Cochrane Database Syst Rev 1:CD005397. https://doi.org/10.1002/14651858.CD005397.pub4

McLaren R, Smith PF, Taylor RL et al (2022) Efficacy of nGVS to improve postural stability in people with bilateral vestibulopathy: a systematic review and meta-analysis. Front Neurosci 16:1010239. https://doi.org/10.3389/fnins.2022.1010239

Meldrum D, Jahn K (2019) Gaze stabilisation exercises in vestibular rehabilitation: review of the evidence and recent clinical advances. J Neurol 266(Suppl 1):11–18. https://doi.org/10.1007/s00415-019-09459-x

Muir SW, Berg K, Chesworth B et al (2010) Quantifying the magnitude of risk for balance impairment on falls in community-dwelling older adults: a systematic review and meta-analysis. J Clin Epidemiol 63(4):389–406. https://doi.org/10.1016/j.jclinepi.2009.06.010

Powell LE, Myers AM (1995) The activities-specific balance confidence (ABC) scale. J Gerontol A Biol Sci Med Sci 50A(1):M28–M34. https://doi.org/10.1093/gerona/50a.1.m28

Rossi-Izquierdo M, Santos-Perez S, Soto-Varela A (2011) What is the most effective vestibular rehabilitation technique in patients with unilateral peripheral vestibular disorders? Eur Arch Otorrinolaringol 268(11):1569–1574. https://doi.org/10.1007/s00405-011-1532-z

Rossi-Izquierdo M, Ernst A, Soto-Varela A et al (2013) Vibrotactile neurofeedback balance training in patients with Parkinson's disease: reducing the number of falls. Gait Posture 37(2):195–200. https://doi.org/10.1016/j.gaitpost.2012.07.002

Rossi-Izquierdo M, Soto-Varela A, Ernst A et al (2016) What could posturography tell us about balance problems in Parkinson's disease? Otol Neurotol 37(9):e326–e331. https://doi.org/10.1097/MAO.0000000000001120

Soto-Varela A, Rossi-Izquierdo M, Del-Rio-Valeiras M et al (2021) Vestibular rehabilitation with mobile posturography as a "low-cost" alternative to vestibular rehabilitation with computerized dynamic posturography, in old people with imbalance: a randomized clinical trial. Aging Clin Exp Res 33(10):2807–2819. https://doi.org/10.1007/s40520-021-01813-2

Sparrer I, Duong Dinh TA, Ilgner J et al (2013) Vestibular rehabilitation using the Nintendo(R) Wii Balance Board—a user-friendly alternative for central nervous compensation. Acta Otolaryngol 133(3):239–245. https://doi.org/10.3109/00016489.2012.732707

Strupp M, Kalla R, Claassen J et al (2011) A randomized trial of 4-aminopyridine in EA2 and related familial episodic ataxias. Neurology 77(3):269–275

Strupp M, Mandala M, Lopez-Escamez JA (2019) Peripheral vestibular disorders: an update. Curr Opin Neurol 32(1):165–173. https://doi.org/10.1097/WCO.0000000000000649

Tinetti ME, Richman D, Powell L (1990) Falls efficacy as a measure of fear of falling. J Gerontol 45(6):P239–P243. https://doi.org/10.1093/geronj/45.6.p239

Tinetti ME, Williams CS, Gill TM (2000) Health, functional, and psychological outcomes among older persons with chronic dizziness. J Am Geriatr Soc 48(4):417–421. https://doi.org/10.1111/j.1532-5415.2000.tb04700.x

Veerbeek JM, van Wegen E, van Peppen R et al (2014) What is the evidence for physical therapy poststroke? A systematic review and meta-analysis. PLoS One 9(2):e87987. https://doi.org/10.1371/journal.pone.0087987

Whitney SL, Sparto PJ (2011) Principles of vestibular physical therapy rehabilitation. NeuroRehabilitation 29(2):157–166. https://doi.org/10.3233/NRE-2011-0690

Whitney SL, Marchetti GF, Schade A et al (2004) The sensitivity and specificity of the timed "up & go" and the dynamic gait index for self-reported falls in persons with vestibular disorders. J Vestib Res 14(5):397–409

Wuehr M, Eder J, Kellerer S et al (2023a) Mechanisms underlying treatment effects of vestibular noise stimulation on postural instability in patients with bilateral vestibulopathy. J Neurol 271:1408. https://doi.org/10.1007/s00415-023-12085-3

Wuehr M, Eder J, Keywan A, Jahn K (2023b) Noisy galvanic vestibular stimulation improves vestibular perception in bilateral vestibulopathy. J Neurol 270(2):938–943. https://doi.org/10.1007/s00415-022-11438-8

Yardley L, Masson E, Verschuur C et al (1992) Symptoms, anxiety and handicap in dizzy patients: development of the vertigo symptom scale. J Psychosom Res 36(8):731–741. https://doi.org/10.1016/0022-3999(92)90131-k

Zwergal A, Strupp M, Brandt T (2019) Advances in pharmacotherapy of vestibular and ocular motor disorders. Expert Opin Pharmacother 20(10):1267–1276. https://doi.org/10.1080/14656566.2019.1610386

Part II

Therapy and Rehabilitation of Peripheral and Central Vestibular Disorders

Peripheral and central vestibular disorders are the major disease entities which lead to dizziness/imbalance. They are clinically most relevant and have largely standardized treatment schemes (in part surgical, e.g., acoustic neuroma or Menière's disease; in part pharmacological, e.g., vestibular migraine or vestibular paroxysmia), but all profit from VRT and coping/counselling.

Peripheral Vestibular Disorders (Labyrinthine Disorders)

3

3.1 Benign Paroxysmal Positional Vertigo (BPPV)

3.1.1 Occurrence and Etiology

Benign paroxysmal positional vertigo (BPPV) is by far the most common vestibular type of vertigo, with an estimated incidence of 64 cases per 100,000 in total and 450/100,000 in the elderly (Bhattacharyya et al. 2008; von Brevern et al. 2007). There is a female-to-male ratio of 2:1 to 3:1. A diagnosis of BPPV is established in 17%–42% of patients with vertigo, depending on age (Hanley et al. 2001). The typical presentation of BPPV consists of brief spinning sensations, usually lasting less than 1 min. Some elderly patients report complaints of prolonged unsteadiness instead of the typical brief vertigo sensation (Batuecas-Caletrio et al. 2013).

BPPV is generally induced by a change in head position with respect to gravity (Furman and Cass 1999). Vertigo frequently develops when a patient gets in or out of bed, rolls over in bed, tilts the head back, or bends forward. The symptoms almost always are worse with changes in head position. Attacks of BPPV are sometimes associated with head trauma (17%), UVL (15%), Meniere's disease (5%), or migraine (5%) (von Brevern et al. 2015). BPPV has also been reported to be associated with osteopenia or osteoporosis and with decreased serum levels of vitamin D independent from age and sex.

> The fundamental pathophysiological process in BPPV involves dislodged otoconia from the macula of the utricular otolith that enters the semicircular canals. When there is a change in the static position of the head with respect to gravity, the otolithic debris moves to a new position within the semicircular canals (canalolithiasis), leading to an increased pressure of the endolymphatic

A. Ernst et al., *Vestibular Therapy and Rehabilitation*, https://doi.org/10.1007/978-3-031-64318-7_3

fluid on the ampullary cupula. Thus, the imagination of a self-rotation is largely enhanced and do not comply with other sensory inputs. This discrepancy in turn induces vertigo.

In some rare cases (below 5%), the otolithic debris is attached to the cupula of one of the canals (cupulolithiasis). Patients with such a kind of BPPV perceive dizziness if the affected cupula is in a non-horizontal position (what is the case most of the time).

BPPV usually arises from the posterior semicircular canal, which is the most gravity-dependent canal. This type of BPPV accounts for 60 to 90% of all cases. BPPV based on the horizontal semicircular canal accounts for 5%–30% of all cases (Parnes et al. 2003). However, the proportion of patients with BPPV based on the horizontal semicircular canal may have been under-estimated especially in the elderly, since involvement at this site is more likely to remit spontaneously than involvement in the posterior semicircular canal (Oghalai et al. 2000). BPPV is rarely based on the anterior semicircular canal (1%–2%), probably because of its uppermost position in the labyrinth, where otolithic debris is unlikely to become trapped during common human behavior (Lopez-Escamez et al. 2005).

Patients with BPPV are at increased risk for falls and impairment in the performance of daily-life activities (Batuecas-Caletrio et al. 2013). Therefore, a speedy and precise diagnose and a proper treatment are of utmost importance. Even if BPPV is the most common vestibular disease, the correct diagnostic procedures are not always performed. Some studies report that only one-third of BPPV patients were diagnosed correctly in general practice (von Brevern et al. 2007).

3.1.2 Diagnostic Procedures

3.1.2.1 Posterior and Anterior Canal BPPV (p-BPPV, a-BPPV)

BPPV is diagnosed by provoking vertigo during positional testing while observing the typical nystagmus. The gold standard for the diagnosis of posterior canal BPPV (p-BPPV) is the Dix-Hallpike maneuver. Mostly, the patient is sitting on an examination couch and is brought fast to a supine position, with the head turned 45° to one side and extended about 20° backward (Fig. 3.1). Thus, the posterior canal is in the movement angel. A positive Dix-Hallpike test is indicated by a combined horizontal-rotational nystagmus. The right side is investigated if the right ear tends to the bottom during the head hanging position. The direction of the nystagmus is counterclockwise if the right side is affected. If the left ear tends to the bottom during the head hanging position, the nystagmus is clockwise if the left side is affected. The nystagmus direction is always indicated by the fast nystagmus phase. A nystagmus latency of up to 30 s is expected during all maneuvers. An important feature of the test is that the nystagmus reverse upon the patient was brought back to a sitting position.

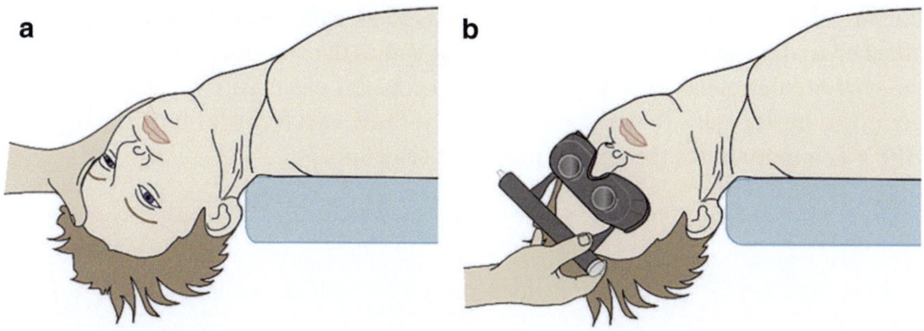

Fig. 3.1 Dix-Hallpike maneuver to detect BPPV(p). (**a**) Fast positioning of the head in reclination (20°) with the tested ear directed to the ground. (**b**) Observation of nystagmus with Frenzel's goggles for at least 1 min. (from Ernst and Basta (2016), with courtesy of the Georg Thieme Verlag KG)

Table 3.1 Differences between positional vertigo of peripheral and central origin

Symptom	Peripheral origin	Central nervous origin
Latency between movement and occurrence of dizziness or nystagmus	0–40 s (mean 7.8 s)	No latency
Duration	Less than 60 s	Several minutes possible
Habituation of symptoms during repetition of provocation	Yes (nearly in 90%)	No
Direction of nystagmus	Fixed direction	Variable direction
Intesity of symptoms and nystagmus	Strong dizziness or vertigo, clear nystagmus, frequently nausea	Mild dizziness or vertigo, less intensive nystagmus, seldom nausea
Reproducability	Inconsistent	Frequently

A vertical (downbeat) nystagmus during the Dix-Hallpike maneuver indicates that the anterior canal could be affected. Further examination is necessary since in a substantial proportion of all cases a vertical nystagmus during the Dix-Hallpike maneuver has a central nervous origin. However, the 75% central origin, reported in some literature is not true as vertical nystagmus also occurs with some stimulations of the SCC hair cells. In general, there is some overlapping between findings which are based on BPPV or central nervous disease. Table 3.1 describes some important differences.

3.1.2.2 Horizontal Canal BPPV (h-BPPV)

A horizontal canal BPPV is diagnosed with the supine roll test. The test is easy to perform since only the head should move fast from one side to the other in a supine position. The test is positive if a horizontal nystagmus appears. The nystagmus is more intense if the movement was performed to the affected ear. It beats either toward the ground (geotropic) or toward the ceiling (apogeotropic). BPPV involving the horizontal canal with geotropic nystagmus is attributed to otolithic debris in the posterior arm while an apogeotropic nystagmus indicates that otolithic debris is attached to the cupula or that is free-floating within the anterior arm of the horizontal semicircular canal. About 75% of all horizontal canal BPPV patients show a geotropic nystagmus. To distinguish between these two forms of horizontal canal, BPPV is important for the correct treatment selection.

During all positional testing, the nystagmus detection should be performed by using Frenzel's goggle or a video goggle to suppress ocular fixation.

3.1.2.3 Additional Anamnestic Features

Beside diagnostic positional maneuvers, patient history is critical for the recognition of BPPV and for classifying the etiology even if the evaluation of a patient with dizziness can be difficult because of the broad etiology and the multiple, nonspecific symptoms especially in the geriatric population. Previous research has identified several items that are useful during history taking of the patient with BPPV, such as the nature of dizziness (i.e., vertigo or light-headedness), the duration of attacks, and the presence and the frequency of associated symptoms (Lindell et al. 2018). Such information is important for predictive models. The purpose of these models is to predict whether a patient presenting with dizziness has BPPV based on the patient's answers to a set of questions. One of these models is the linear prediction, which has shown promising results in the prediction of BPPV (Britt et al. 2018). However, one very important factor in the patient file for the prediction of BPPV is the history of BPPV since the annual rate of BPPV recurrence is approximately 15% (Nunez et al. 2000).

3.1.3 Treatment Options

BPPV often resolves without treatment. The spontaneous remission of BPPV episodes is likely because of the fact that endolymph, based on its low content of ionized calcium (20 μM), can in some cases dissolve dislodged otoconia (Zucca et al. 1998). The median interval between the onset of symptoms and spontaneous resolution in untreated patients is nearly 1 week when the horizontal canal is affected and 2 weeks when the posterior canal is affected (Imai et al. 2005). To reduce the patient's distress, BPPV can be well-treated with repositioning procedures. Nearly 75% of BPPV patients have no further complaints after a first repositioning procedure, 94% after a second and approximately 98% after a third treatment. Home training could be helpful for a fully relief from symptoms. The selection of the specific repositioning maneuver depends on the affected canal. Therefore, a careful diagnostic is very important for the treatment outcome.

3.1.3.1 Posterior Canal BPPV (p-BPPV)

Upon a positive Dix-Hallpike test with a detected horizontal/rotational nystagmus mostly the Epley's canalith-repositioning maneuver is applied to flush mobile otolithic debris out of the posterior canal and back into the vestibule. The Epley maneuver is divided in 4 steps (Fig. 3.2a). Step 1 (B) brings the patient in a supine position, with the head turned 45° to one side and extended about 20° backward (as during the Dix-Hallpike maneuver). The affected side tends to the bottom during the head hanging position. The nystagmus should be monitored. In step 2 (C), the head is turned to the opposite side. Step 3 is performed by asking the patient to lay on the contralateral shoulder (to the affected ear) and positioning the head parallel to the floor. The last step (D) directs the patient's head to face the floor. Each next step should always be performed for at least 30 s and after the decay of the nystagmus or vertigo. If the maneuver was successful, the patient should not show any nystagmus after he is brought in a sitting position. The use of a vibrator on the mastoid of the affected side while Epley's maneuver is being performed has little evidence (Hunt et al. 2012).

For patients who have difficulties extending the neck, the Semont maneuver can be used to treat BPPV affecting the posterior canal. The patient is rapidly swung during the maneuver from lying on the affected side to lying on the unaffected side within approximately 1 second (Fig. 3.2b). Both Epley's and Semont's maneuvers may be repeated several times until no nystagmus is elicited. A modification (Semont plus) has been recently described (Strupp et al. 2021). Success rate of Epley's maneuvers seems to be much higher than those of Semont's maneuvers. Success rate of Semont plus is higher than Semont. After the treatment, it is helpful for patients to sit still, in an upright position, for about 15 min and to walk then cautiously.

3.1.3.2 Anterior Canal BPPV (a-BPPV)

BPPV affecting the anterior canal should be treated if a vertical (downbeat) nystagmus was detected during the Dix-Hallpike maneuver, and a central origin could be excluded. An effective repositioning maneuver was described by Yacovino et al. (Yacovino et al. 2009). During the maneuver (Fig. 3.3), the patient is rapidly laid down from a sitting position on the examination bed to a head hanging at an angle of at least 30° over the end of the bed for a duration of 30–180 s (the longer is the better). The head should then be lifted quickly to touch the patient's chest for additional 30–180 s. Afterwards the patient comes back to a seated position. The maneuver may be repeated several times until the nystagmus disappeared.

3.1.3.3 Horizontal Canal BPPV (h-BPPV)

A horizontal canal BPPV with a geotropic nystagmus can be treated by the Barbeque rotation or the Gufoni's maneuver. The success rate after a single application of the latter is much higher (38% vs. 89%) (Korres et al. 2011). The barbecue rotation techniques work by negative inertia. They are done performing abrupt rotations of the patient's head in steps of 90° toward the healthy side while supine, thus moving the debris in the direction opposite to the head rotation. The head is rotated three

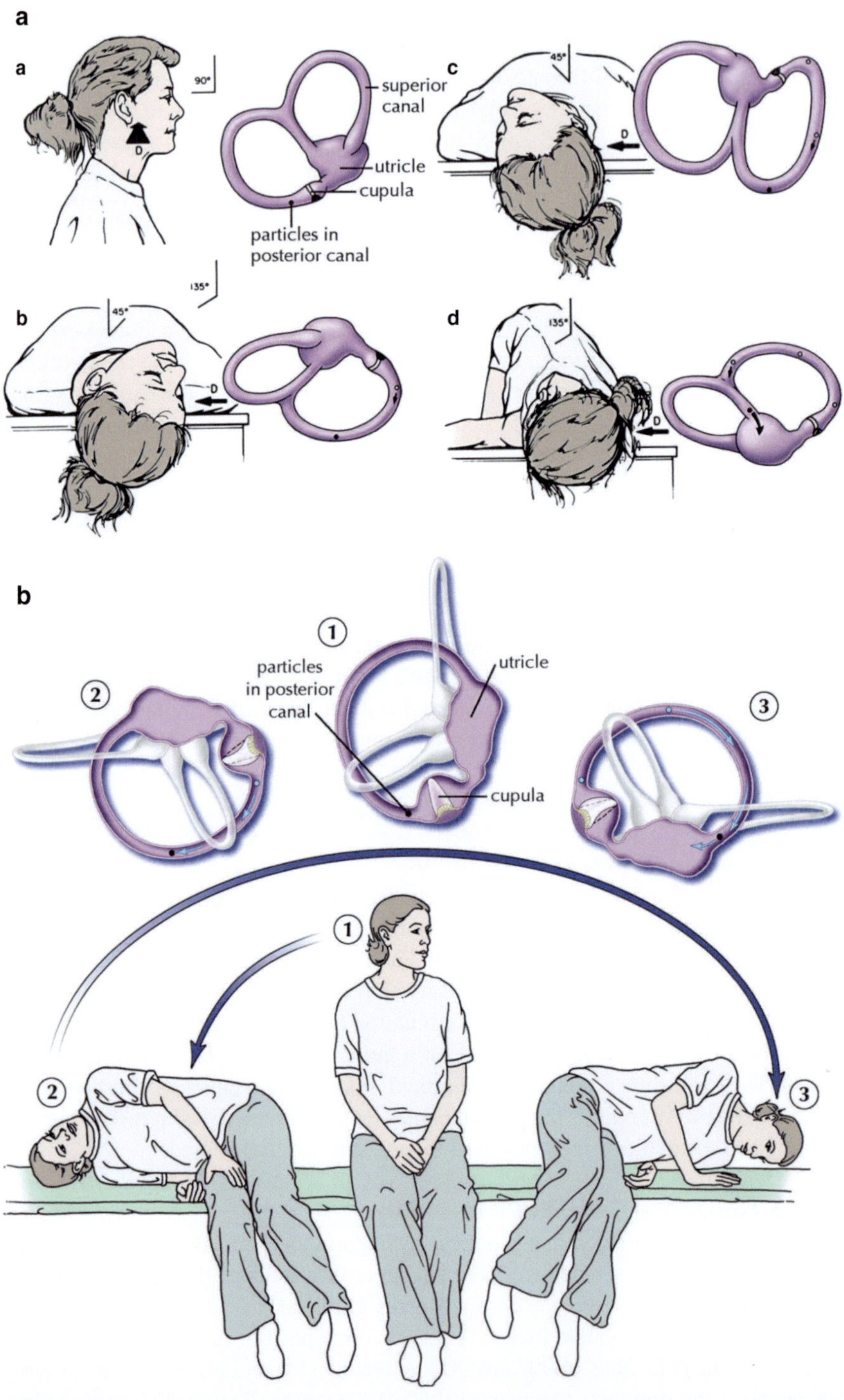

Fig. 3.2 Epley's (**a**) and Semont's (**b**) maneuver to treat p-BPPV (from Parnes et al. 2003, with courtesy of the Canadian Medical Association)

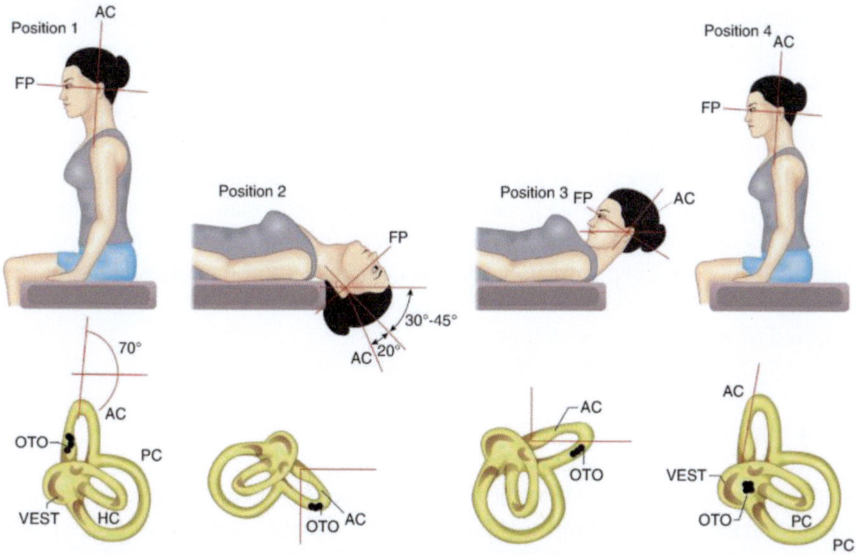

Fig. 3.3 Yacovino maneuver to treat a-BPPV (from Albernaz et al. (2019), with courtesy of Springer Nature)

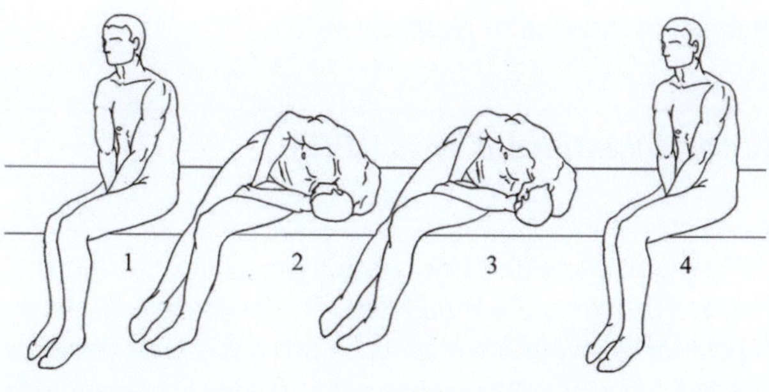

Fig. 3.4 Gufoni's maneuver to treat h-BPPV (from Albernaz et al. (2019), with courtesy of Springer Nature)

times toward the healthy side to provide an overall 270° rotation. To apply the Gufoni's maneuver (Fig. 3.4), the patient quickly lies down on the side of the unaffected ear and remains in this position for 1–2 min, until the evoked nystagmus subsides. The head is then quickly rotated 45° toward the floor and kept in this position for another 2 min before the patient return to an upright position.

Treatment of horizontal canal BPPV with an apogeotropic nystagmus involves maneuvers designed to detach the otolithic debris from the cupula or to move the debris from the anterior arm of the horizontal canal to the posterior arm. Possible strategies include headshaking in the horizontal plane for 15 s or modified Gufoni's maneuver. The modified Gufoni's maneuver seems to be somewhat more effective (62% and 73%, respectively). During the maneuver, the patient sits upright, looking straight head, and then quickly lies down on the affected side and remains in this position for 1–2 min. Then the head is quickly turned 45° toward the ceiling and is held in this position for 2 min. Now the otolithic debris that is lying near or is adherent to the cupula in the anterior arm of the horizontal canal is moved to a more posterior position. Here it may fall into the vestibule or can be removed with the use of Gufoni's maneuver for horizontal canal BPPV with geotropic nystagmus, in which the head is turned in step 3 toward the floor, as described above (Fig. 3.4). In patients which do not respond to any of the repositioning maneuvers some surgical procedures have been described, such as neurectomies of the ampullary nerve and canal occlusion. In some untreatable patients, a stenosis of the semicircular canal by a mass of otoconia could be observed in MRI-reconstructions and successfully removed by a surgical intervention.

3.1.4 Medication

Medications are mainly used to relieve severe nausea or vomiting in the acute phase. The pharmacological treatment of BPPV with vestibular suppressive drugs is not effective and thus not a substitute for repositioning maneuvers (Hain and Yacovino 2005). However, the maneuvers sometimes are only tolerated after symptomatic drug treatment. Although reduced vitamin D levels have been reported among persons with BPPV (Jeong et al. 2013), it is unknown whether vitamin D supplementation reduces the risk of incident or recurrent BPPV.

3.2 Unilateral Vestibular Loss (UVL)

The clinical picture of acute UVL (synonym: acute vestibular syndrome, AVS) is characterized by a disabling vertigo (patients usually have to remain in a supine position for hours) with sudden onset (seconds–minutes), accompanied by nausea, vomiting, head motion intolerance, and instability in stance and gait conditions (Fetter 2016). No hearing loss. Idiopathic origin (e.g., viral, microcirculatory possible) (Fetter 2016). Diagnostic criteria have recently been published (Strupp et al. 2022).

3.2.1 Diagnostic Findings and Differential Diagnosis

Patients show a spontaneous, peripheral horizontal and rotatory nystagmus with quick phases toward the unaffected ear, which slowly cessates (over days to weeks) and can be suppressed by visual fixation. Head impulse test (HIT) shows the deficit of the lateral SCC. This can be confirmed by caloric testing and/or video-HIT. Ischemic stroke (e.g., PICA infarction) is the most relevant differential diagnosis (mostly normal HIT). Other differential diagnoses include Ramsay Hunt syndrome (Varicella zoster), monosymptomatic vestibular attack in VM or MD, AN, etc. (CT/MRI is advised for exclusion) (Fetter 2016).

3.2.2 Time Course and Therapy

Two thirds of all patients fully compensate the functional deficit of the lateral SCC, and the HIT becomes normal after some weeks (Curthoys and Halmagyi 1995). The compensatory process has a static phase (1–3 weeks) when the patient can move around again and a dynamic phase when the patient can perform more complex tasks (e.g., riding a bike, playing squash) (Allum and Honegger 2016). If the subjective complaints (nausea, vomiting) are overwhelming, vestibular suppressants (e.g., dimenhydrinate) can be given for relief within the first few days (see Table 2.2 for details). Acute medical therapy includes the administration of corticosteroids (different dosage regimes and application modes possible) or phytotherapeutics (Lindner et al. 2019) (Fig. 3.5). Antiviral drugs do not show convincing effects in the idiopathic UVL (in contrast to Ramsay Hunt syndrome).

Home exercises are recommended (Figs. 2.10, 2.11, 2.12) in the first (static) phase, supported by a physiotherapist if required (twice daily). They should consist of gaze, stance, and gait exercises when the patient can get up alone from supine and start to move around. Gaze exercises can be done in bed or in a sitting position. Thereafter, in the dynamic phase of compensation (after about 2–3 weeks), specialized vestibular rehabilitation (VRT) should be performed (see Chap. 2) with emphasis on the residual vestibular deficit (SCC, otolith organs).

Acute onset, diagnostics completed (UVL)

↓

Medical treatment, antemetics ($\approx$1-5 days),
after leaving bed: stance exercises

↓

Gaze stabilizing exercises, stance and gait exercises
(initially with a PT, followed by home training for 2–3 weeks)

↓

Re-evaluation of the patient (any scc/otolith deficits left ?)

↙ ↘

Full compensation: no more VR, normal life-style (incl sports)	residual deficit: individualized VR (for some weeks/months)

Fig. 3.5 Diagnostic/therapeutic procedure in patients with UVL (*PT* Physiotherapist, *VRT* Vestibular rehabilitation therapy)

3.2.3 Risk and Pitfalls

One-third of the patients after UVL do not compensate, the HIT shows a deficit of the lateral SCC after several months, in some patients additional functional losses (other SCC, saccule, utricle) can be found subsequently (Halmagyi et al. 2010).

They should undergo a cardiovascular workup (including a search for an irregular blood-pressure regulation—e.g., non- or inverted dipping or obstructive sleep apnea) which can reveal pathophysiological patterns preventing a central compensation by neuroplasticity. In those cases, special medication is required.

Elderly patients (with diabetes, microcirculatory disorders, cardiovascular risk factors, obesity) require long-term PT by activation (general recommendation: 1 h exercise/day, if only walking) (Ohara et al. 2020).

3.3 Bilateral Vestibular Loss (BVL)

BVL must be excluded in all patients with gait instability and dizziness that is only present when moving, i.e., during standing and walking. It is common in the elderly (presbyvestibulopathy) (Jahn et al. 2019; Agrawal et al. 2019). BVL is often combined with peripheral neuropathy and sometimes combined with both neuropathy and cerebellar dysfunction (Cortese et al. 2021). Most patients have an incomplete loss of peripheral vestibular function (Zingler et al. 2007).

Patients with bilateral vestibulopathy present with gait instability, worsening in darkness, and on uneven ground. They do not experience spinning vertigo, nausea, or vomiting. Most patients suffer from chronic progressive deficits. They all need balance training.

3.3.1 Diagnostic Findings and Differential Diagnosis

Patients report dizziness and balance problems during walking that become worse in darkness (or with eyes closed) and on uneven ground (e.g., when walking on forest trails) (Jahn 2019; Schniepp et al. 2021). Due to the loss of function of the vestibular ocular reflex (VOR), some patients report apparent moving of the surroundings (oscillopsia) when moving the head during walking and while driving on bumpy roads (Zingler et al. 2007). The hallmark finding on clinical examination is a bilateral pathological head impulse test (HIT) (Strupp et al. 2017). The loss of function for the semicircular canals can be quantified by the video HIT for high frequencies and by calorics (only lateral canal) for low frequencies. Involvement of otolith organs can be tested by VEMPs. Dynamic visual acuity (DVA) is usually impaired. Patients have no symptoms at rest. The main differential diagnosis are other sensory deficits, in particular peripheral neuropathy (distal hypaesthesia and normal HIT). BHV is often overseen, as the presentation is less dramatic compared to acute UVL. Etiology of BVL is unknown (idiopathic) in about 1/3 of cases. Common specific aetiologies are vitamin B12 deficiency, bilateral Menière's disease, or inner ear autoimmunity (in younger patients) (Zingler et al. 2007; Jahn et al. 2015).

3.3.2 Time Course and Therapy

BVL is in most cases slowly progressive over years. Elderly persons often develop a mild BVL in parallel to hearing loss (presbyacusis and presbyvestibulopathy) (Jahn et al. 2019). Therapy can be in some cases directed to the specific etiology (e.g., vitamin B12 supplementation or steroids in autoimmune disease). Patients have an increased risk to fall (Wuehr et al. 2022). All patients need symptomatic treatment by VRT with intensive training of stance and gait conditions. Recently, restoration of vestibular function by invasive surgery became available (vestibular implant) (van den Berg et al. 2011). This is so far only an option for selected cases with nearly complete loss of function and hearing loss (because of the risk of hearing loss due to surgery). An emerging treatment option is non-invasive stimulation by subtle direct currents (white noise galvanic vestibular stimulation = nGVS, see Chap. 2) (Eder et al. 2022; Wuehr et al. 2023).

3.3.3 Risks and Pitfalls

Many cases of BVL are overseen and not diagnosed correctly. Although patients with balance problems should get balance and gait training anyway, the correct diagnosis opens the way to a more specific therapy (VRT, see Figs. 2.10 and 2.11).

> About 40% of BVL patients fall repetitively due to the sensory deficit (Schlick et al. 2016; Wuehr et al. 2022). As the vestibular deficit can at least partly be compensated by other sensory systems (vision, proprioception), most patients can get around sufficiently with VRT. Patients that cannot tolerate the deficit at all often show signs of an accompanying functional dizziness.

3.4 Endolymphatic Hydrops and Menière's Disease (MD)

3.4.1 Diagnostic Findings and Differential Diagnosis

Since MD is a progressive disorder which apoptotically destroys the auditory and vestibular sensory cells (Ishiyama et al. 2015), there are no uniform neurotological findings. Apart from the progressive SNHL, usually the horizontal SCC is impaired during attacks (spontaneous nystagmus to the affected ear) (Hirai et al. 2017). Over time (years—decades), the SCC and the otolith organs are destroyed (Duwel et al. 2005; Hannigan et al. 2019; van Tilburg et al. 2016). Finally, when the utricle is not more intact, sudden drop attacks with a loss of postural control, but no unconsciousness (Tumarkin crises) can occur (Tumarkin 1936).

The most important differential diagnosis is vestibular migraine (VM), but VM patients have a normal hearing (Lempert et al. 2012). On the other hand, 1/3 of all MD patients develop VM over time (subsequently or in parallel) (Murofushi et al. 2018). SCDS can mimic MD. Rare entities as most important differential diagnosis are endolymphatic sac tumors/delayed endolymphatic hydrops.

3.4.2 Time Course and Therapy

The attack-like vertigo is treated in its beginning with diet and drugs (ICON) (Fig. 3.6), later stages are treated surgically (endolymphatic sac surgery, occlusion of the lateral SCC, in Tumarkin crisis labyrinthectomy in combination with cochlear implantation for auditory rehabilitation) (Nevoux et al. 2018; Doobe et al. 2015). In between, gentamicin and/or prednisone can be applied as intratympanic therapy. Since the individual decline of the balance performance is highly variable, the patients should be advised to be physically active to stabilize their postural performance (Gottshall et al. 2010). When single deficits (SCC/otolith organs) become clinically apparent, they should be addressed by deficit-specific exercises (see Chap. 2).

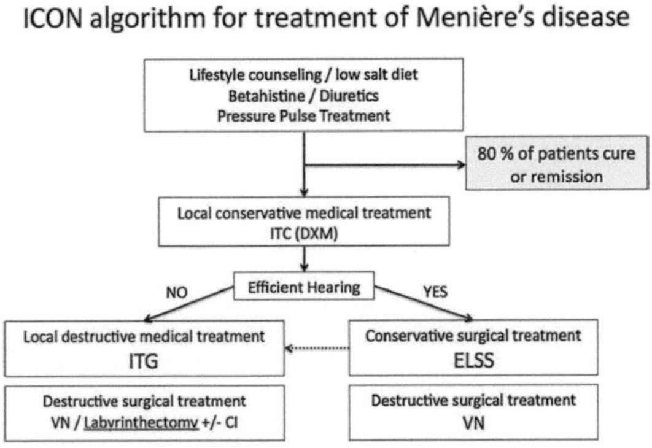

Fig. 3.6 International consensus (ICON) on the treatment of Menière's disease (Nevoux et al. 2018) (*ITC* Intratympanic therapy with dexamethasone—DXM, *ITG* Intratympanic gentamicin, *ELSS* Endolymphatic shunt surgery, *VN* Vestibular neurectomy, *CI* Cochlear implantation), comment: VN is usually replaced nowadays by surgical occlusion of the lateral SCC (Charpiot et al. 2010)

One-third of the patients have a bilateral MD. This bears the risk of developing BVL (Frejo et al. 2016). Chemical or surgical destruction of the vestibular organ to bring relief because of the vertiginous attacks should be limited to one ear, if possible. The auditory rehabilitation of the SNHL (hearing aids, CI) is important, too, to improve spatial orientation (Doobe et al. 2015).

3.4.3 Risk and Pitfalls

Elderly patients (with diabetes, microcirculatory disorders, cardiovascular risk factors, obesity) require long-term PT by activation (general recommendation: 1 h exercise/day) (Ohara et al. 2020). Common comorbidities (e.g., autoimmune disorders, fibromyalgia) should be considered and treated accordingly (Frejo et al. 2016).

3.5 Dehiscence Syndromes of the Semicircular Canals (SCDS/PCDS)

The present chapter is limited to the descriptions of dehiscence of the superior and posterior SCCs. Well-known for many decades have been the dehiscence/fistulae of the lateral SCC, usually induced by chronic otitis media/cholesteatoma which are known to have dizziness as a leading symptom.

The clinical picture of SCDS is highly variable (Ward et al. 2017). From no symptoms to massive MD-like attacks and from normal hearing—mixed HL-near-total deafness, anything goes. The clinical picture depends largely on the size of the dehiscence and on comorbidities, particularly the parallel occurrence of VM (Ward et al. 2017). The patients frequently complain additionally of autophony, Tullio's phenomenon, and oscillopsia upon fast movements (e.g., running). PCDS has a less prominent clinical picture and males fewer clinical complaints.

3.5.1 Diagnostic Findings and Differential Diagnosis

The audiological findings are variable (see above). In the beginning, c/oVEMP changes are most characteristic (Hunter et al. 2017). The most important diagnostic criterion is an open superior SCC on HR-CT scans of the petrous bone (1.5–2 mm slice thickness) (Ernst et al. 2016). All other diagnostic signs (e.g., Hennebert's) are not reliable enough. Due to the specificity of the structural abnormality (open

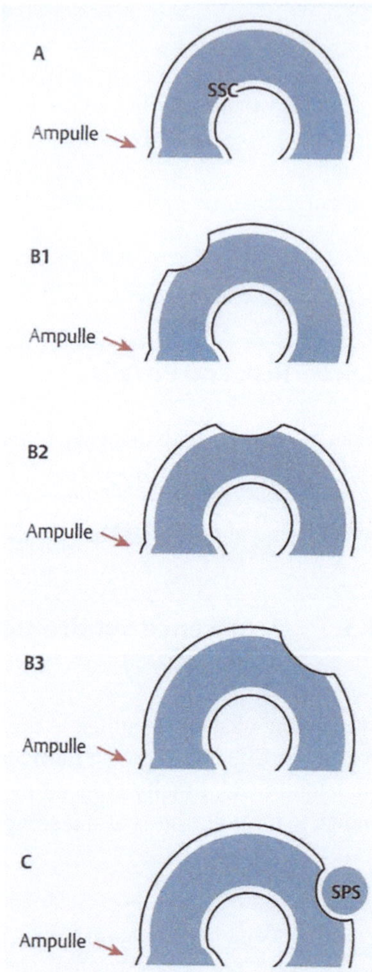

Fig. 3.7 SCDS at different locations of the SCC (A: normal; B1–3: different locations at the eminentia arcuata; C: SCDS by the superior petrous sinus)

superior and/or posterior SCC), there are no real differential diagnoses possible (Fig. 3.7). However, SCDS can mimic MD, sudden HL.

3.5.2 Time Course and Therapy

The time course is unpredictable. In some patients, the disorder is clinically silent until a blunt head trauma triggers vertiginous complaints (Brodsky et al. 2018). Antivertiginous drugs can reduce those complaints (see Chap. 2), but finally, the surgical occlusion of the superior SCC is the method-of-choice in patients with severe vertigo. VRT is helpful particularly after surgery to speed up compensation/recovery. iNFT has the highest success rate (Basta et al. 2011).

3.5.3 Risks and Pitfalls

The most critical decision is when to perform surgery and in whom. Patients with larger dehiscence, additional VM and elderly patients (65+) have a poorer outcome (Gioacchini et al. 2016). VRT is most helpful after surgery; home exercises should be continued for at least 3 months (Carender and Grzesiak 2018). BPPV is most frequent within the next 24 months after surgery (5% of all patients after surgical repair) (Xie et al. 2017).

References

Agrawal Y, Van de Berg R, Wuyts F et al (2019) Presbyvestibulopathy: diagnostic criteria consensus document of the classification committee of the Barany Society. J Vestib Res 29(4):161–170. https://doi.org/10.3233/VES-190672

Albernaz PLM, e Maia FZ, Carmona S, Cal RVR, Zalazar G (2019) The New Neurotology-A Comprehensive Clinical Guide. Spinger Nature, Switzerland

Allum JH, Honegger F (2016) Recovery times of stance and gait balance control after an acute unilateral peripheral vestibular deficit. J Vestib Res 25(5–6):219–231. https://doi.org/10.3233/VES-150561

Basta D, Rossi-Izquierdo M, Soto-Varela A et al (2011) Efficacy of a vibrotactile neurofeedback training in stance and gait conditions for the treatment of balance deficits: a double-blind, placebo-controlled multicenter study. Otol Neurotol 32(9):1492–1499. https://doi.org/10.1097/MAO.0b013e31823827ec

Batuecas-Caletrio A, Trinidad-Ruiz G, Zschaeck C et al (2013) Benign paroxysmal positional vertigo in the elderly. Gerontology 59(5):408–412. https://doi.org/10.1159/000351204

van den Berg R, Guinand N, Stokroos RJ et al (2011) The vestibular implant: quo vadis? Front Neurol 2:47

Bhattacharyya N, Baugh RF, Orvidas L et al (2008) Clinical practice guideline: benign paroxysmal positional vertigo. Otolaryngol Head Neck Surg 139(5 Suppl 4):S47–S81. https://doi.org/10.1016/j.otohns.2008.08.022

von Brevern M, Radtke A, Lezius F et al (2007) Epidemiology of benign paroxysmal positional vertigo: a population based study. J Neurol Neurosurg Psychiatry 78(7):710–715. https://doi.org/10.1136/jnnp.2006.100420

von Brevern M, Bertholon P, Brandt T et al (2015) Benign paroxysmal positional vertigo: Diagnostic criteria. J Vestib Res 25(3–4):105–117. https://doi.org/10.3233/VES-150553

Britt CJ, Ward BK, Owusu Y et al (2018) Assessment of a statistical algorithm for the prediction of benign paroxysmal positional vertigo. JAMA Otolaryngol Head Neck Surg 144(10):883–886. https://doi.org/10.1001/jamaoto.2018.1657

Brodsky JR, Shoshany TN, Lipson S et al (2018) Peripheral vestibular disorders in children and adolescents with concussion. Otolaryngol Head Neck Surg 159(2):365–370. https://doi.org/10.1177/0194599818770618

Carender WJ, Grzesiak M (2018) Vestibular rehabilitation following surgical repair for Superior Canal Dehiscence Syndrome: a complicated case report. Physiother Theory Pract 34(2):146–156. https://doi.org/10.1080/09593985.2017.1374491

Charpiot A, Rohmer D, Gentine A (2010) Lateral semicircular canal plugging in severe Meniere's disease: a clinical prospective study about 28 patients. Otol Neurotol 31(2):237–240. https://doi.org/10.1097/MAO.0b013e3181ca85a2

Cortese A, Curro R, Vegezzi E et al (2021) Cerebellar ataxia, neuropathy and vestibular areflexia syndrome (CANVAS): genetic and clinical aspects. Pract Neurol 22:14. https://doi.org/10.1136/practneurol-2020-002822
Curthoys IS, Halmagyi GM (1995) Vestibular compensation: a review of the oculomotor, neural, and clinical consequences of unilateral vestibular loss. J Vestib Res 5(2):67–107
Doobe G, Ernst A, Ramalingam R et al (2015) Simultaneous labyrinthectomy and cochlear implantation for patients with single-sided Meniere's disease and profound sensorineural hearing loss. Biomed Res Int 2015:457318. https://doi.org/10.1155/2015/457318
Duwel P, Walther LE, Ilgner J et al (2005) Time-dependent vestibular function loss of semicircular canals and otolith organs in Meniere's disease. Laryngorhinootologie 84(8):589–593. https://doi.org/10.1055/s-2005-861248
Eder J, Kellerer S, Amberger T et al (2022) Combining vestibular rehabilitation with noisy galvanic vestibular stimulation for treatment of bilateral vestibulopathy. J Neurol 269(11):5731–5737. https://doi.org/10.1007/s00415-022-11033-x
Ernst A, Todt I, Wagner J (2016) Dehiscence syndromes : diagnosis and treatment. HNO 64(11):790–796. https://doi.org/10.1007/s00106-016-0255-2
Ernst, Basta (2016) Gleichgewichtsstörungen. Thieme, Stuttgart
Fetter M (2016) Acute unilateral loss of vestibular function. Handb Clin Neurol 137:219–229. https://doi.org/10.1016/B978-0-444-63437-5.00015-7
Frejo L, Soto-Varela A, Santos-Perez S et al (2016) Clinical subgroups in bilateral Meniere disease. Front Neurol 7:182. https://doi.org/10.3389/fneur.2016.00182
Furman JM, Cass SP (1999) Benign paroxysmal positional vertigo. N Engl J Med 341(21):1590–1596. https://doi.org/10.1056/NEJM199911183412107
Gioacchini FM, Alicandri-Ciufelli M, Kaleci S et al (2016) Outcomes and complications in superior semicircular canal dehiscence surgery: a systematic review. Laryngoscope 126(5):1218–1224. https://doi.org/10.1002/lary.25662
Gottshall KR, Topp SG, Hoffer ME (2010) Early vestibular physical therapy rehabilitation for Meniere's disease. Otolaryngol Clin N Am 43(5):1113–1119. https://doi.org/10.1016/j.otc.2010.05.006
Hain TC, Yacovino D (2005) Pharmacologic treatment of persons with dizziness. Neurol Clin 23(3):831–853, vii. https://doi.org/10.1016/j.ncl.2005.01.012
Halmagyi GM, Weber KP, Curthoys IS (2010) Vestibular function after acute vestibular neuritis. Restor Neurol Neurosci 28(1):37–46. https://doi.org/10.3233/RNN-2010-0533
Hanley K, O'Dowd T, Considine N (2001) A systematic review of vertigo in primary care. Br J Gen Pract 51(469):666–671
Hannigan IP, Welgampola MS, Watson SRD (2019) Dissociation of caloric and head impulse tests: a marker of Meniere's disease. J Neurol 268:431. https://doi.org/10.1007/s00415-019-09431-9
Hirai C, Yamamoto Y, Takeda T et al (2017) Nystagmus at the onset of vertiginous attack in Meniere's disease. Otol Neurotol 38(1):110–113. https://doi.org/10.1097/MAO.0000000000001255
Hunt WT, Zimmermann EF, Hilton MP (2012) Modifications of the Epley (canalith repositioning) manoeuvre for posterior canal benign paroxysmal positional vertigo (BPPV). Cochrane Database Syst Rev (4):CD008675. https://doi.org/10.1002/14651858.CD008675.pub2
Hunter JB, Patel NS, O'Connell BP et al (2017) Cervical and ocular VEMP testing in diagnosing superior semicircular canal dehiscence. Otolaryngol Head Neck Surg 156(5):917–923. https://doi.org/10.1177/0194599817690720
Imai T, Ito M, Takeda N et al (2005) Natural course of the remission of vertigo in patients with benign paroxysmal positional vertigo. Neurology 64(5):920–921. https://doi.org/10.1212/01.WNL.0000152890.00170.DA
Ishiyama G, Lopez IA, Sepahdari AR et al (2015) Meniere's disease: histopathology, cytochemistry, and imaging. Ann N Y Acad Sci 1343:49–57. https://doi.org/10.1111/nyas.12699
Jahn K (2019) The aging vestibular system: dizziness and imbalance in the elderly. Adv Otorhinolaryngol 82:143–149. https://doi.org/10.1159/000490283

Jahn K, Kressig RW, Bridenbaugh SA et al (2015) Dizziness and unstable gait in old age: etiology, diagnosis and treatment. Deutsches Arzteblatt Int 112(23):387–393. https://doi.org/10.3238/arztebl.2015.0387

Jahn K, Freiberger E, Eskofier BM et al (2019) Balance and mobility in geriatric patients : assessment and treatment of neurological aspects. Z Gerontol Geriatr 52(4):316–323. https://doi.org/10.1007/s00391-019-01561-z

Jeong SH, Kim JS, Shin JW et al (2013) Decreased serum vitamin D in idiopathic benign paroxysmal positional vertigo. J Neurol 260(3):832–838. https://doi.org/10.1007/s00415-012-6712-2

Korres S, Riga MG, Xenellis J et al (2011) Treatment of the horizontal semicircular canal canalithiasis: pros and cons of the repositioning maneuvers in a clinical study and critical review of the literature. Otol Neurotol 32(8):1302–1308. https://doi.org/10.1097/MAO.0b013e31822f0bc5

Lempert T, Olesen J, Furman J et al (2012) Vestibular migraine: diagnostic criteria. J Vestib Res 22(4):167–172. https://doi.org/10.3233/VES-2012-0453

Lindell E, Finizia C, Johansson M et al (2018) Asking about dizziness when turning in bed predicts examination findings for benign paroxysmal positional vertigo. J Vestib Res 28(3–4):339–347. https://doi.org/10.3233/VES-180637

Lindner M, Gosewisch A, Eilles E et al (2019) Ginkgo biloba extract EGb 761 improves vestibular compensation and modulates cerebral vestibular networks in the rat. Front Neurol 10:147. https://doi.org/10.3389/fneur.2019.00147

Lopez-Escamez JA, Gamiz MJ, Fernandez-Perez A et al (2005) Long-term outcome and health-related quality of life in benign paroxysmal positional vertigo. Eur Arch Otorrinolaringol 262(6):507–511. https://doi.org/10.1007/s00405-004-0841-x

Murofushi T, Tsubota M, Kitao K et al (2018) Simultaneous presentation of definite vestibular migraine and definite Meniere's disease: overlapping syndrome of two diseases. Front Neurol 9:749. https://doi.org/10.3389/fneur.2018.00749

Nevoux J, Barbara M, Dornhoffer J et al (2018) International consensus (ICON) on treatment of Meniere's disease. Eur Ann Otorhinolaryngol Head Neck Dis 135(1S):S29–S32. https://doi.org/10.1016/j.anorl.2017.12.006

Nunez RA, Cass SP, Furman JM (2000) Short- and long-term outcomes of canalith repositioning for benign paroxysmal positional vertigo. Otolaryngol Head Neck Surg 122(5):647–652. https://doi.org/10.1016/S0194-5998(00)70190-2

Oghalai JS, Manolidis S, Barth JL et al (2000) Unrecognized benign paroxysmal positional vertigo in elderly patients. Otolaryngol Head Neck Surg 122(5):630–634. https://doi.org/10.1067/mhn.2000.105415

Ohara A, Yasuhiro M, Mochizuki F et al (2020) Effects of using cane and vestibular rehabilitation on the walking function in elderly patients with dizziness. Auris Nasus Larynx 48:571. https://doi.org/10.1016/j.anl.2020.10.010

Parnes LS, Agrawal SK, Atlas J (2003) Diagnosis and management of benign paroxysmal positional vertigo (BPPV). CMAJ 169(7):681–693

Schlick C, Schniepp R, Loidl V, Wuehr M, Hesselbarth K, Jahn K (2016) Falls and fear of falling in vertigo and balance disorders: A controlled cross-sectional study. J Vestib Res. 25(5-6):241–51 https://doi.org/10.3233/VES-150564. PMID: 26890425.

Schniepp R, Huppert A, Decker J et al (2021) Fall prediction in neurological gait disorders: differential contributions from clinical assessment, gait analysis, and daily-life mobility monitoring. J Neurol 268(9):3421–3434. https://doi.org/10.1007/s00415-021-10504-x

Strupp M, Kim JS, Murofushi T et al (2017) Bilateral vestibulopathy: diagnostic criteria consensus document of the classification Committee of the Barany Society. J Vestib Res 27(4):177–189. https://doi.org/10.3233/VES-170619

Strupp ML, Straumann D, Helmchen C (2021) Nystagmus: diagnosis, topographic anatomical localization and therapy. Klin Monatsbl Augenheilkd 238(11):1186–1195. https://doi.org/10.1055/a-1525-0030

Strupp M, Bisdorff A, Furman J et al (2022) Acute unilateral vestibulopathy/vestibular neuritis: Diagnostic criteria. J Vestib Res 32(5):389–406. https://doi.org/10.3233/VES-220201

van Tilburg MJ, Herrmann BS, Guinan JJ Jr et al (2016) Serial cVEMP testing is sensitive to disease progression in Meniere patients. Otol Neurotol 37(10):1614–1619. https://doi.org/10.1097/MAO.0000000000001213

Tumarkin A (1936) The otolithic catastrophe: a new syndrome. Br Med J 2(3942):175–177. https://doi.org/10.1136/bmj.2.3942.175

Ward BK, Carey JP, Minor LB (2017) Superior canal dehiscence syndrome: lessons from the first 20 years. Front Neurol 8:177. https://doi.org/10.3389/fneur.2017.00177

Wuehr M, Decker J, Schenkel F et al (2022) Impact on daily mobility and risk of falling in bilateral vestibulopathy. J Neurol 269:5746. https://doi.org/10.1007/s00415-022-11043-9

Wuehr M, Eder J, Keywan A et al (2023) Noisy galvanic vestibular stimulation improves vestibular perception in bilateral vestibulopathy. J Neurol 270(2):938–943. https://doi.org/10.1007/s00415-022-11438-8

Xie Y, Sharon JD, Pross SE et al (2017) Surgical complications from superior canal dehiscence syndrome repair: two decades of experience. Otolaryngol Head Neck Surg 157(2):273–280. https://doi.org/10.1177/0194599817706491

Yacovino DA, Hain TC, Gualtieri F (2009) New therapeutic maneuver for anterior canal benign paroxysmal positional vertigo. J Neurol 256(11):1851–1855. https://doi.org/10.1007/s00415-009-5208-1

Zingler VC, Cnyrim C, Jahn K et al (2007) Causative factors and epidemiology of bilateral vestibulopathy in 255 patients. Ann Neurol 61(6):524–532

Zucca G, Valli S, Valli P et al (1998) Why do benign paroxysmal positional vertigo episodes recover spontaneously? J Vestib Res 8(4):325–329

4 Central Vestibular Disorders

4.1 Vestibular Schwannoma/Acoustic Neuroma (AN)

The clinical picture of ANs is highly variable depending on the localization of this benign tumor (intra–/extra-intrameatal, intracochlear). Primary symptom is mostly a unilateral sudden hearing loss (SNHL) and/or tinnitus, and larger tumors are correlated with vertigo of different characteristics and extent (Malhotra et al. 2009).

4.1.1 Diagnostic Findings and Differential Diagnosis

The SNHL is the leading symptom in AN, when the tumor grows fast, different neurotological symptoms accompany the SNHL. Calorics and/or HIT evidence SCC losses, otolith disorders follow (Brown et al. 2019). MRI is advised in all sudden HL episodes to exclude AN (Fig. 4.1).

4.1.2 Time Course and Therapy

The small intracanalicular tumors are under MRI follow-up (watch & scan) to evidence a possible growth. Larger tumors should undergo resection and/or irradiation (when the balance is compromised/sudden falls occur and/or the facial nerve function is impaired).

Isolated losses of balance function (SCC/utricle/saccule) during follow-up (see above) should undergo a balance training directed at the specific deficit (see Figs. 2.10, 2.11, 2.12). After surgical resection or radiotherapy, the vestibular nerve is usually lost. Patients then have a high fall's risk and an impaired embodied spatial cognition (Deroualle et al. 2019). They should be definitely rehabilitated as patients with an uncompensated UVL and counselled in addition (fall prevention) (Fig. 4.2).

A. Ernst et al., *Vestibular Therapy and Rehabilitation*, https://doi.org/10.1007/978-3-031-64318-7_4

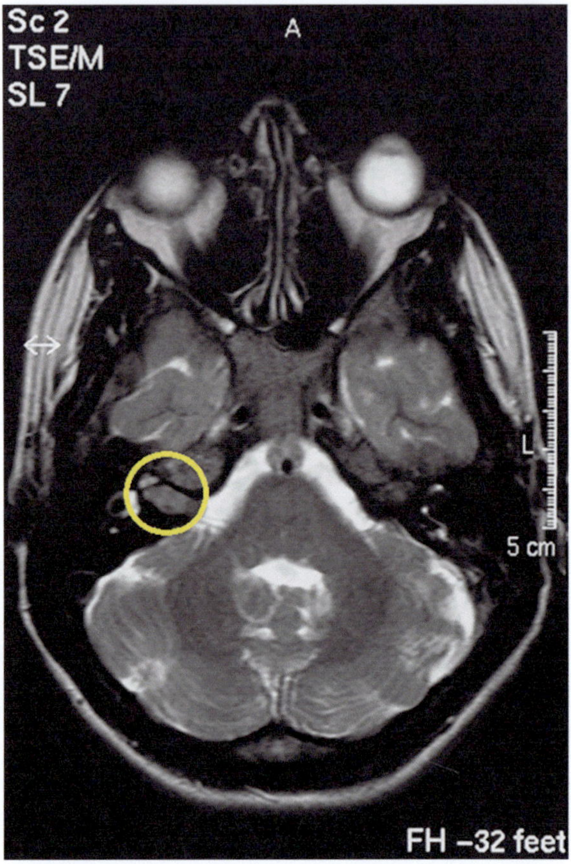

Fig. 4.1 Acoustic neuroma (VN) with intra–/extrameatal extension (MRI scan)

(pre-hab)

↓

AN therapy
(surgical resection, radiotherapy)

↓

Neurotological diagnostics
(to define vestibular deficits)

↙ ↘

Partial VN loss
(Specific VR exercises)

complete VN loss (deafferentiation)
(gaze/gait exercises/PT/VR)

Fig. 4.2 Neurorehabilitation approach in AN-patients after therapy (microsurgical resection/radiotherapy) with/without pre-hab (see text) (superior/inferior VN—vestibular nerve; VRT—vestibular rehabilitation; PT—physical therapy)

4.1.3 Risks and Pitfalls

After surgical resection of the tumor, the deafferentation of the peripheral vestibular organ is most critical for stance and gait, but the preoperative vestibular impairment by the tumor is abolished by its removal so that even elderly patients can have an improved balance performance after surgery (Gauchard et al. 2012). However, the best outcome for a compensated balance function can be expected for those patients who had been physically active before surgery (Gauchard et al. 2012). In addition, a so-called PRE-HAB could help to overcome the critical postop period, i.e., before surgery, certain exercises should be trained after preop treatment with gentamicin (Tjernstrom et al. 2018) (see Figs. 2.10, 2.11, 2.12). After radiosurgery, the same problem occurs, but with a latency of about 6 months (and should be dealt with equally) (Kim et al. 2020).

4.2 Vestibular Migraine (VM)

Migraine is common in the general population (up to 25% of women and 15% of men). A substantial proportion of patients suffering from migraine also reports at least some dizziness and balance problems. VM affects up to 1% of the general population (Lempert et al. 2012). Diagnostic criteria for VM have first been proposed in 1999 (Dieterich and Brandt 1999) and 2001 (Neuhauser et al. 2001) and at least consented by the Bárány-Society in 2012 and by the International Headache Society in 2013 (Lempert et al. 2012; Headache Classification Committee of the International Headache Society (IHS) 2013). VM affects younger patients more often than aged ones and can be difficult to diagnose because of the lack of specific tests.

Vestibular migraine is the most common cause of spontaneously occurring vertigo spells. It is most common in young patients (children, adolescents, and young adults). The mainstay of treatment is prophylactic by physical activity and—if needed prophylactic drug therapy (see Table 2.2).

4.2.1 Diagnostic Findings and Differential Diagnosis

The diagnostic criteria for VM are published and available in the most recent update online (Lempert et al. 2012). In short: Patients suffering from vestibular migraine have attacks with a duration between 5 min and 72 h (in MD attacks with spinning vertigo lasting less than 5 h are more typical). Patients should have the history of classical migraine (headache) and some typical migraine features (headache quality, photo- and phonophobia). Vestibular symptoms during the attack can be spinning vertigo, positional vertigo, visually induced vertigo or had motion induced vertigo. Patients during the attack can show nystagmus, postural imbalance, nausea, and vomiting. Between attacks there often is a mild central ocular motor syndrome (e.g., saccadic pursuit). The main differential diagnosis of VM is Menière's disease (MD) because both disorders can have similar durations of attacks. To make the correct diagnosis is not difficult when V presents typically (vertigo, dizziness, postural imbalance, sensitivity to light and noise, nausea, vomiting; all without any signs of peripheral vestibular dysfunction). However, there are many patients that fall between both diagnoses, i.e., it is not unusual to have both disease entities in one patient since there is an overlap (Murofushi et al. 2018).

Laboratory testing between attacks is mostly unremarkable. Peripheral vestibular dysfunction occurs but is by far not typical. There is a high comorbidity for motion sickness, depression, and anxiety disorders (Lahmann et al. 2015; Strupp et al. 2018).

4.2.2 Time Course and Therapy

There is a lifelong predisposition for migraine in susceptible subjects. Many patients have a positive family history. Over the lifespan, there are often periods with lots of migraine attacks (headache, vertigo, and dizziness) followed by other periods with only single or no attacks at all (Langhagen et al. 2015). Time spans with headache only can be followed by time spans with only vestibular symptoms. Younger patients are more often affected from migraine (childhood, adolescence, younger adult life) (Filippopulos et al. 2017; Langhagen et al. 2016; Jahn et al. 2015). The time course often shows a spontaneous improvement and undulation over time.

Attacks can be treated in the same way as classical migraine headache attacks (medication to reduce nausea, pain medication, rest in a dark room). However, the most important aspect of treatment is prophylactic to prevent attacks. The first choice for prophylactic treatment is the complete set of non-pharmaceutical approaches. Among these regular aerobic endurance training (at least three times 30 min per week) and the learning and use of relaxation techniques are most effective. In cases where non-pharmacological approaches are not sufficient, the next option would be the prophylactic pharmaceutical treatment (see Table 2.2) using, for example, beta-blockers, calcium antagonists, antiepileptic drugs, or tricyclic antidepressants (amitriptyline). Vestibular rehabilitation therapy (VRT) is sometimes helpful. However, as vestibular migraine is an episodic disorder, it is not that often needed. There is in the typical cases no loss of vestibular function and no progressive deficit over time. This means that patients should get their physical activity to a high level, but mostly do not need special balance training.

4.2.3 Risks and Pitfalls

VM is an episodic central vestibular disorder. Due to the episodic character, it is not likely to oversee other central disorders that usually present with continuous symptoms (e.g., posterior fossa brain tumors). Migraine is a lifelong disorder. It changes its activity, however, dependent on, e.g., the hormonal status. In this way, the maturation in adolescence as well as hormonal transitions in later adulthood often changes the character of migraine. VM can therefore be present in a phase of life and later the patient suffers from headache migraine or from isolated visual auras.

An MRI should be taken in cases with ocular motor signs that exceed the known mild ocular motor abnormalities often seen in vestibular migraine. In the differential diagnosis to Menière's disease (which is usually accompanied by a hearing loss), it is sometimes necessary to treat the more likely diagnosis first and switch to the less likely in case of no effect.

4.3 Vestibular Paroxysmia (VP)

Vestibular paroxysmia is caused by neuro-vascular cross compression at the vestibulo-cochlear nerve and characterized by short attacks (seconds) of spinning or swaying vertigo (Hufner et al. 2008). A classification of the disorder has been consented by the Bárány-Society in 2016 (Strupp et al. 2016). Response to pharmacological treatment is part of these criteria. The disorder also occurs in children and adolescents (Lehnen et al. 2015).

> Vestibular paroxysmia accounts for about 5% of cases in dizziness clinics. It is characterized by very short attacks (seconds) occurring spontaneously. The easiest way to make the diagnosis is to start drug treatment. Attacks will disappear or at least get reduced within days.

4.3.1 Diagnostic Findings and Differential Diagnosis

Diagnosis is suspected in all patients reporting short attacks of vertigo or dizziness lasting less than 1 min. Typical attacks occur spontaneously but can sometimes also be provoked by headshaking or hyperventilation (Hufner et al. 2008). Cochlear symptoms, in particular tinnitus, can occur. Figure 4.3 shows the location of vascular cross compression as the pathophysiology of the disorder.

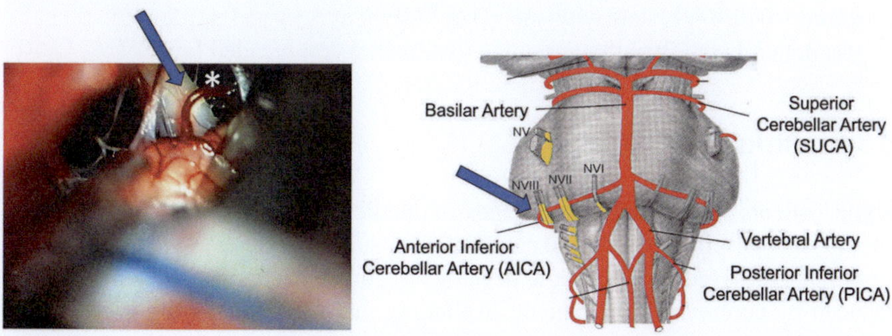

Fig. 4.3 Susceptible area of the vestibular-cochlear nerve (asterisk: AICA loop) at the root entry zone and other cranial nerves where vascular cross compression causes paroxysmal symptoms

Other disorders presenting with short spells of vertigo and dizziness can usually be differentiated by taking a careful history. BPPV is always provoked by head and body movements, orthostatic dizziness occurs when standing up from a lying or sitting position, and perilymph fistula and dehiscence syndrome are associated with changes of middle ear pressure (coughing, sneezing, Valsalva maneuvre) or by specific sounds. The most difficult differential diagnosis might be a functional dizziness that sometimes goes along with short dizziness attacks. The latter are usually presenting as light-headedness and not as vertigo. They are always part of a broader combination of different complaints. It can also be difficult to differentiate VP from brainstem paroxysms as they occur, e.g., in multiple sclerosis.

In laboratory tests, a mild unilateral vestibular loss can be documented. The neuro-vascular cross compression can be visualized on MRI with focus on CSF spaces (CISS or FIESTA sequence) (Strupp et al. 2013). As many asymptomatic patients also show a cross compression, the response to pharmacological treatment with sodium channel blockers (see Table 2.2) is at least as relevant as the finding on MRI (Brandt et al. 2016).

4.3.2 Time Course and Therapy

Treatment response to sodium channel blocking substances is fast and therefore a test treatment is important to make the diagnosis (see Table 2.2). The classical substances used are carbamazepine or oxcarbazepine, but also lacosamide or lamotrigine will work (Strupp et al. 2019). Patients should be advised to document their attack frequency in a diary. The course is usually benign in the sense that attacks disappear under treatment. However, they often come back when tapering down the medication and the effect of medication sometimes becomes worse with time. Surgery (Jannetta) is an alternative that is not often needed (Strupp et al. 2013).

> As vestibular paroxysmia only shows short attacks, vestibular rehabilitation therapy is usually not needed. Making the diagnosis and initiating treatment can prevent the secondary development of functional dizziness. Some patients with BVL start with short paroxysmal attacks and develop the bilateral deficit later. They then need the treatment recommended for BVL.

4.3.3 Risks and Pitfalls

Some patients need increased dosages of medication over time. Those patients should be counselled as potential candidates for surgery (microvascular decompression, Jannetta surgery). The risk to develop a secondary functional dizziness can be reduced by counselling the patient, explaining the nature of the disorder, and by starting drug treatment early.

4.4 Vestibular Stroke

In up to 15% of patients presenting with acute vertigo, symptoms are caused by stroke (Jahn et al. 2020). Most of these strokes are in the posterior circulation and include ischemic lesions in the brainstem (e.g., Wallenberg's syndrome) and in the cerebellum. About 10% of strokes are missed at first contact in the emergency department (Tarnutzer et al. 2017). This is true for transitory ischemic attacks (TIA) when clinical signs already disappeared on presentation at the emergency room. Patients after short episodes of vertigo have a 50-fold increased risk to be readmitted with stroke within the next week (Atzema et al. 2016). A classification for vascular vertigo has recently been published (Kim et al. 2022). This classification helps to define central syndromes and further differentiate them from the typical peripheral AVS.

Recent evidence shows that stroke is more common as a cause for acute vertigo and dizziness than thought in the past. Taking vascular risk factors into account in dizzy patients can help to predict the likelihood of a serious etiology (stroke) in the individual patient (e.g., ABCD2-score) (Edlow et al. 2018).

4.4.1 Diagnostic Findings and Differential Diagnosis

The key to diagnosis in vestibular stroke is the careful clinical examination. The detection of signs and symptoms pointing to central involvement excludes the peripheral vestibular differential diagnosis. For the acute vestibular syndrome (AVS), the differential diagnosis is between acute UVL and brainstem/cerebellar stroke (Jahn et al. 2020). In this situation, the HINTS criteria apply, which means that a normal head impulse test, skew deviation, and/or direction change of nystagmus on lateral gaze point to central origin of the AVS (Kattah et al. 2009). However, many patients with vestibular strokes have transient symptoms, gait unsteadiness and lateropulsion, double vision, or dizziness with nausea. Whenever these symptoms appear for the first time and the clinical examination does not elucidate the origin, an MRI of the brain should be made. Affected areas are shown in Fig. 4.4. However, the gold standard is the combination of clinical signs and MRI as the MRI alone misses up to 30% of vestibular strokes (Zwergal and Dieterich 2020).

4.4.2 Time Course and Therapy

As soon as a stroke is suspected, cerebral bleeding should be excluded (CT scan) and intravenous thrombolysis can be initiated when the patient presents less than 4.5 h after symptom onset and has relevant deficits. In all other cases, the focus is on identification of risk factors for and etiology of the stroke to initiate the adequate secondary prophylactic treatment. Most patients will do best with acetylsalicylic

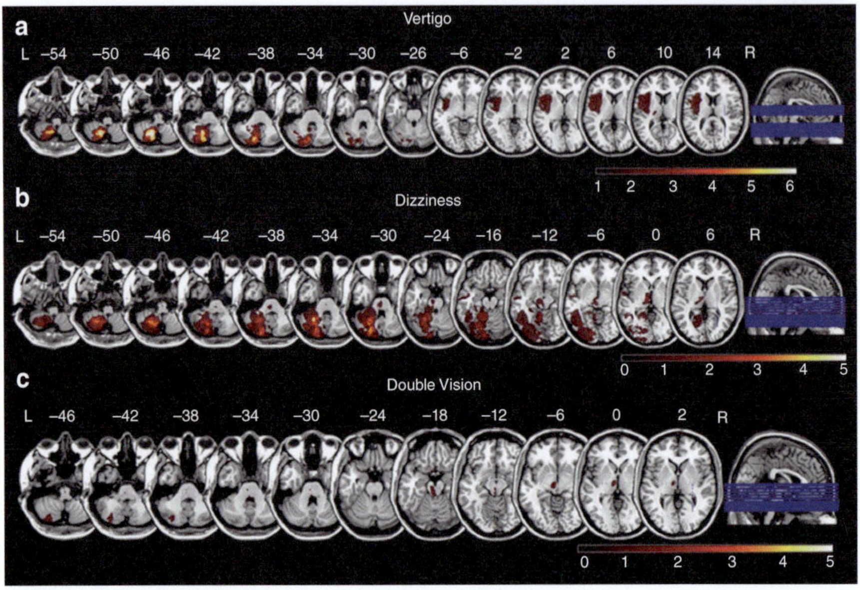

Fig. 4.4 Lesion distribution in stroke patients with the leading symptoms vertigo, dizziness, or double vision (Zwergal et al. 2020)

acid (ASS) and a statin on the long run. Patients with atrial fibrillation need anticoagulation.

Patients with persistent deficits should receive rehabilitation including balance training and exercises for combined head and eye movements. In some cases, this will be a classical VRT. In many patients, additional elements of training are needed. Stroke patients improve over time, and vestibular strokes in general have a good prognosis (Schuhbeck et al. 2022).

4.4.3 Risks and Pitfalls

There is a high risk of recurrent strokes after a first event (Zwergal and Dieterich 2020). The best prophylaxis is the compliance with the medication and the reduction of risk factors. Strokes with dizziness can present in many ways. It remains essential to be able to perform and interpret the detailed ocular motor, vestibular, and neurological examination.

References

Atzema CL, Grewal K, Lu H et al (2016) Outcomes among patients discharged from the emergency department with a diagnosis of peripheral vertigo. Ann Neurol 79(1):32–41. https://doi.org/10.1002/ana.24521

Brandt T, Strupp M, Dieterich M (2016) Vestibular paroxysmia: a treatable neurovascular cross-compression syndrome. J Neurol 263(Suppl 1):S90–S96. https://doi.org/10.1007/s00415-015-7973-3

Brown CS, Peskoe SB, Risoli T Jr et al (2019) Associations of video head impulse test and caloric testing among patients with vestibular schwannoma. Otolaryngol Head Neck Surg 161(2):324–329. https://doi.org/10.1177/0194599819837244

Deroualle D, Borel L, Tanguy B et al (2019) Unilateral vestibular deafferentation impairs embodied spatial cognition. J Neurol 266(Suppl 1):149–159. https://doi.org/10.1007/s00415-019-09433-7

Dieterich M, Brandt T (1999) Episodic vertigo related to migraine (90 cases): vestibular migraine? J Neurol 246(10):883–892

Edlow JA, Gurley KL, Newman-Toker DE (2018) A new diagnostic approach to the adult patient with acute dizziness. J Emerg Med 54(4):469–483. https://doi.org/10.1016/j.jemermed.2017.12.024

Filippopulos FM, Albers L, Straube A et al (2017) Vertigo and dizziness in adolescents: risk factors and their population attributable risk. PLoS One 12(11):e0187819. https://doi.org/10.1371/journal.pone.0187819

Gauchard GC, Lion A, Perrin PP et al (2012) Influence of age on postural compensation after unilateral deafferentation due to vestibular schwannoma surgery. Laryngoscope 122(10):2285–2290. https://doi.org/10.1002/lary.23497

Headache Classification Committee of the International Headache Society (IHS) (2013) The International Classification of Headache Disorders, 3rd edition (beta version). Cephalalgia 33(9):629–808. https://doi.org/10.1177/0333102413485658

Hufner K, Barresi D, Glaser M et al (2008) Vestibular paroxysmia: diagnostic features and medical treatment. Neurology 71(13):1006–1014

Jahn K, Langhagen T, Heinen F (2015) Vertigo and dizziness in children. Curr Opin Neurol 28(1):78–82. https://doi.org/10.1097/WCO.0000000000000157

Jahn K, Kreuzpointner A, Pfefferkorn T et al (2020) Telling friend from foe in emergency vertigo and dizziness: does season and daytime of presentation help in the differential diagnosis? J Neurol 267(Suppl 1):118–125. https://doi.org/10.1007/s00415-020-10019-x

Kattah JC, Talkad AV, Wang DZ et al (2009) HINTS to diagnose stroke in the acute vestibular syndrome: three-step bedside oculomotor examination more sensitive than early MRI diffusion-weighted imaging. Stroke 40(11):3504–3510

Kim G, Hullar TE, Seo JH (2020) Comparison of balance outcomes according to treatment modality of vestibular schwannoma. Laryngoscope 130(1):178–189. https://doi.org/10.1002/lary.27830

Kim JS, Newman-Toker DE, Kerber KA et al (2022) Vascular vertigo and dizziness: diagnostic criteria. J Vestib Res 32(3):205–222. https://doi.org/10.3233/VES-210169

Lahmann C, Henningsen P, Brandt T et al (2015) Psychiatric comorbidity and psychosocial impairment among patients with vertigo and dizziness. J Neurol Neurosurg Psychiatry 86(3):302–308. https://doi.org/10.1136/jnnp-2014-307601

Langhagen T, Albers L, Heinen F et al (2015) Period prevalence of dizziness and vertigo in adolescents. PLoS One 10(9):e0136512. https://doi.org/10.1371/journal.pone.0136512

Langhagen T, Landgraf MN, Huppert D et al (2016) Vestibular migraine in children and adolescents. Curr Pain Headache Rep 20(12):67. https://doi.org/10.1007/s11916-016-0600-x

Lehnen N, Langhagen T, Heinen F et al (2015) Vestibular paroxysmia in children: a treatable cause of short vertigo attacks. Dev Med Child Neurol 57(4):393–396. https://doi.org/10.1111/dmcn.12563

Lempert T, Olesen J, Furman J et al (2012) Vestibular migraine: diagnostic criteria. J Vestib Res 22(4):167–172. https://doi.org/10.3233/VES-2012-0453

Malhotra PS, Sharma P, Fishman MA et al (2009) Clinical, radiographic, and audiometric predictors in conservative management of vestibular schwannoma. Otol Neurotol 30(4):507–514. https://doi.org/10.1097/MAO.0b013e31819d3465

Murofushi T, Tsubota M, Kitao K et al (2018) Simultaneous presentation of definite vestibular migraine and definite Meniere's disease: overlapping syndrome of two diseases. Front Neurol 9:749. https://doi.org/10.3389/fneur.2018.00749

Neuhauser H, Leopold M, von Brevern M et al (2001) The interrelations of migraine, vertigo, and migrainous vertigo. Neurology 56(4):436–441

Schuhbeck F, Strobl R, Conrad J et al (2022) Determinants of functioning and health-related quality of life after vestibular stroke. Front Neurol 13:957283. https://doi.org/10.3389/fneur.2022.957283

Strupp M, von Stuckrad-Barre S, Brandt T et al (2013) Teaching neuroimages: compression of the eighth cranial nerve causes vestibular paroxysmia. Neurology 80(7):e77. https://doi.org/10.1212/WNL.0b013e318281cc2c

Strupp M, Lopez-Escamez JA, Kim JS et al (2016) Vestibular paroxysmia: Diagnostic criteria. J Vestib Res 26(5–6):409–415. https://doi.org/10.3233/VES-160589

Strupp M, Brandt T, Huppert D et al (2018) Prevalence of motion sickness in various vestibular disorders: a study on 749 patients. J Neurol 265(Suppl 1):95–97. https://doi.org/10.1007/s00415-018-8961-1

Strupp M, Elger C, Goldschagg N (2019) Treatment of vestibular paroxysmia with lacosamide. Neurol Clin Pract 9(6):539–541. https://doi.org/10.1212/CPJ.0000000000000610

Tarnutzer AA, Lee SH, Robinson KA et al (2017) ED misdiagnosis of cerebrovascular events in the era of modern neuroimaging: a meta-analysis. Neurology 88(15):1468–1477. https://doi.org/10.1212/WNL.0000000000003814

Tjernstrom F, Fransson PA, Kahlon B et al (2018) PREHAB vs. REHABILITATION—presurgical treatment in vestibular schwannoma surgery enhances recovery of postural control better than postoperative rehabilitation: retrospective case series. J Vestib Res 27(5–6):313–325. https://doi.org/10.3233/VES-170626

Zwergal A, Dieterich M (2020) Vertigo and dizziness in the emergency room. Curr Opin Neurol 33(1):117–125. https://doi.org/10.1097/WCO.0000000000000769

Zwergal A, Mohwald K, Salazar Lopez E et al (2020) A prospective analysis of lesion-symptom relationships in acute vestibular and ocular motor stroke. Front Neurol 11:822. https://doi.org/10.3389/fneur.2020.00822

Part III

Therapy and Rehabilitation of Vertigo and Dizziness as Major Symptoms in Different Etiologies

Vertigo and dizziness are most prominent complaints (apart from headache and back pain) in the Western world. The aging Western societies have a substantial share of elderly people. When they acquire age-related dizziness (presbyvestibulopathy), this makes them prone to falls. But dizziness in general can be an accompanying symptom of other, very different medical conditions.

Dizziness over the Life-Span

5

Migraine-related syndromes account for about 40% of diagnoses in children with vertigo and dizziness. Somatoform vertigo (with normal findings on clinical examination) is common in adolescence. Central vestibular syndromes related to serious causes (e.g., tumor of the posterior intracranial fossa) are rare and can easily be detected by careful clinical examination. Most vertigo syndromes in childhood are benign and can be effectively treated.

5.1 Dizziness in Childhood and Adolescence

Children may find it hard to report on their complaints. It might be difficult to say how long spells of vertigo and dizziness last, as well as what provokes or accompanies them. Because children are inexperienced in describing their vestibular concerns as dizziness or vertigo, clinical and laboratory tests become more important (Yang et al. 2023).

5.1.1 Taking the History in Children

History taking should focus on the points summarized in Table 5.1. It is of some importance to differentiate spinning from to-and-for vertigo, as well as episodic and sustained vertigo. Patients should always be asked about any headache and cochlear symptoms (e.g., hearing loss, tinnitus).

A. Ernst et al., *Vestibular Therapy and Rehabilitation*,
https://doi.org/10.1007/978-3-031-64318-7_5

Table 5.1 Taking the history in dizzy children and adolescents

• Ask for	Comments
• Type of vertigo/ dizziness	Spinning vertigo, imbalance, gait instability, lightheadedness
• Duration of symptoms	Attacks lasting • Seconds–Minutes (e.g., Vestibular Paroxysmia, Benign Paroxysmal Positional Vertigo = BPPV) • Minutes–Hours (e.g., Menière's Disease, Vestibular Migraine) • Days–Weeks (e.g., Labyrinthitis, Vestibular Neuritis) • Months–Years (e.g., Cerebellar Ataxia, Stroke)
• Provoking factors	Change of head position (e.g., BPPV) Coughing, sneezing (e.g., Perilymph Fistula) Specific foods (e.g., Vestibular Migraine)
• Additional symptoms	Hearing loss or pressure in the ear (e.g., Menière's Disease Headache (e.g., Vestibular Migraine)

5.1.2 Neuro-otological Examination in Children

Clinical examination of peripheral and central vestibular function in children is possible from very young age on (about 6 months) (Fife et al. 2000). It must include ocular motor testing, head impulses, and balance tests. Because peripheral vestibular nystagmus is suppressed by visual fixation, it is mandatory to prevent fixation (with Frenzel's goggles) when searching for spontaneous nystagmus. Neuronal circuits for ocular motor and vestibular function develop within the first year of life and can be reliably tested, even in toddlers. The head impulse test for horizontal vestibulo-ocular reflex function is easily performed at the bedside or in the office (Jahn et al. 2015b). Video-oculography systems with inertial sensors for synchronized recording of head and eye velocity allow quantification of vestibulo-ocular gains and are well tolerated. Reponses to caloric irrigation of the ears have been successfully recorded in children as young as 1 year of age. Rotational testing has some advantages over caloric testing, if the primary goal is to determine the presence or absence of vestibular function. Caloric testing is superior for quantification of the deficit. Vertigo is less intense in rotational chair testing than during caloric testing. Small children can sit in an adult's lap during the rotational chair testing (Jahn 2016). The examiner looks for optokinetic nystagmus during rotation. The vestibular response of the horizontal semicircular canal is best observed when the chair is stopped after 5–10 rotations at constant velocity (about 180 deg./s). The quick phases of the vestibular nystagmus beat opposite to the direction of rotation (e.g., to the left after stopping a chair rotation to the right). The nystagmus duration should be symmetric for left and right rotations. Further, body sway can be quantified using force plates or accelerometers as an objective measure for postural imbalance. Brain MRI should be considered in all patients presenting with subacute central vestibular signs to exclude brain tumors, encephalitis, malformation, and others.

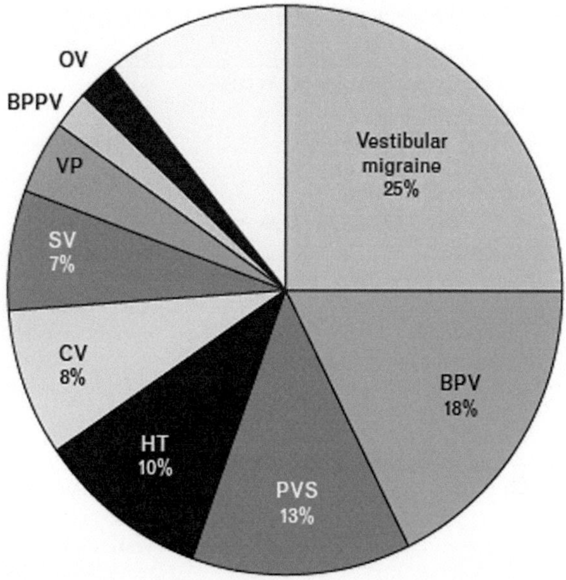

Fig. 5.1 Frequency distribution among dizzy children (Jahn et al. 2015b)

5.1.3 Differential Diagnosis of Vertigo and Dizziness in Children

The spectrum of diagnoses is like that in adults, but the incidence rates are different (Filippopulos et al. 2017). Figure 5.1 shows the distribution of diagnoses pooled from different centers reporting on more than 2000 patients. Migraine is the most common cause of recurrent vertigo in children, i.e., approximately 40% of vertigo syndromes in children are related to migraine (e.g., benign paroxysmal vertigo of childhood, vestibular migraine) (Langhagen et al. 2016). Psychosomatic disorders are a common cause of chronic vertigo in adolescents and children older than 10 years. The most common cause of vertigo in adults, benign paroxysmal positional vertigo (BPPV), is less frequent in children, but it still accounts for a substantial proportion of diagnoses. Motion sickness is a frequent and relevant problem in children aged 4–10 years. Children with a few rare congenital syndromes (e.g., CHARGE syndrome) present with bilateral vestibular failure. Vestibular epilepsy is a rarity: only single-proven cases have been reported worldwide (Jahn 2016) (Tables 5.2 and 5.3).

5.1.3.1 Benign Paroxysmal Vertigo

Benign paroxysmal vertigo of childhood is the most common cause of episodic vertigo in children between 2 and 6 years of age (Abu-Arafeh and Russell 1995; van de Berg et al. 2021), usually as the result of any head trauma. The clinical presentation is characterized by short episodes of vertigo or dizziness (seconds to minutes), often associated with nystagmus and postural imbalance. In some cases, headache, nausea, and vomiting are also present. Cochlear symptoms (hearing loss or tinnitus)

Table 5.2 Therapy of peripheral vestibular disorders in children

Clinical syndrome	Therapeutic options
Benign Paroxysmal Positional Vertigo (BPPV)	
• Posterior canal (up to 90%) • Horizontal canal (about 10%) • Anterior canal (<1%)	Specific release maneuvre
Acute Unilateral Vestibular Loss	
• Labyrinthitis – viral – bacterial (in meningitis) – serous (otitis) – autoimmune (e.g., Cogan's syndrome) • Traumatic • Vestibular Neuritis	General measures: • Day 1–3: symptomatic treatment with vestibular suppressants (e.g., dimenhydrinate) • Early mobilization to support central compensation • Therapy based on the specific cause: **viral:** in Zoster oticus: acyclovir 3 × 5 mg/kg/day **bacterial:** antibiotics **serous:** treatment of otitis (antibiotics) **autoimmune:** prednisolone, 1 mg/kg/day, dose reduction depends on response **vestibular neuritis:** prednisolone, 1 mg/kg/day, reduction by 20% every 3rd day
Vestibular Paroxysmia	Carbamazepine, 2–6 mg/kg/day Oxcarbazepine, 4–8 mg/kg/day
Perilymph Fistula	
• From middle to inner ear (posttraumatic, postinfectious, cholesteatoma) • From inner ear to the middle cranial fossa (superior canal dehiscence)	• Therapy of underlying disease • Conservative therapy with avoidance of provocation • Surgery infrequently necessary
Bilateral Vestibulopathy	
• congenital • postinfectious (meningitis) • toxic (aminoglycosides) • malnutrition (vitamin B12, folic acid) • autoimmune • degenerative (Cerebellar Ataxia) • neoplastic (e.g., Bilateral Vestibular Schwannoma) • idiopathic	• Balance training to support sensory substitution by visual and somatosensory systems • Treatment of the specific cause

are not typical. Children do not show any signs of vestibular dysfunction between attacks. The frequency of attacks can widely differ. The disorder can manifest in the first 2 years of life and usually disappears spontaneously around age 6. Later in life, typical migraines may develop; in these cases, there is often a family history of classical migraine. Paroxysmal torticollis and periodic vomiting (other migraine equivalents) also occur with vertigo and dizziness, with similar presentation as benign paroxysmal vertigo of childhood. Because of the benign nature of these disorders, drug therapy is rarely necessary.

Table 5.3 Therapy of central vestibular disorders in children

Clinical syndrome	Therapeutic options
Central lesion	
• Neoplastic (e.g., cerebellar/ brainstem tumor) • Degenerative/hereditary (e.g., Cerebellar Ataxia, Episodic Ataxia) • Inflammatory (e.g., brainstem encephalitis) • Vascular (e.g., malformation) • Traumatic (e.g., brainstem concussion) • Epileptic (e.g., vestibular aura)	Therapy based on the aetiology **Episodic ataxia type II:** • Acetazolamide, 5–10 mg/kg/day • 4-Aminopyridine, 5 mg (qd, bid, tid, experience in children based on single cases) **Downbeat/Upbeat nystagmus:** • 4-Aminopyridine (see above)
Migraine related	
Benign Paroxysmal Vertigo of childhood (BPV)	Drug prophylaxis rarely necessary because of the benign course; prophylaxis in cases with frequent or severe attacks (falls) possible (see below)
Vestibular Migraine, Basilar type migraine (Migraine with brainstem aura)	Avoidance of provoking factors (alimentary, stress, lack of sleep); relaxation techniques; sufficient physical activity (sports); sufficient fluid intake
	Drug prophylaxis recommended with frequent (≥3/month) and/or severe attacks (>72 h) • Magnesium aspartate, 200–400 mg/day • Propranolol, 1–2 mg/kg/day • Metoprololsuccinate, 0.5–1 mg/kg/day • Topiramate, 1–2 mg/kg/day • Amitriptyline, 0.5–1 mg/kg/day • Valproic acid, 10–20 mg/kg/day • Levetiracetam, 20–30 mg/kg/day
Motion Sickness	Behavioural prophylaxis by visual control/ feedback (looking out of the car), avoidance of heavy meals before travelling, sufficient fresh air, distraction Drug prophylaxis: • Dimenhydrinate, 1–2 mg/kg, every 6 h

5.1.3.2 Vestibular Migraine in Children and Adolescents

In several clinical case series, more than 50% of dizzy children also have headache irrespective of the final diagnosis (van de Berg et al. 2021). Typical for vestibular migraine are episodic attacks of rotatory or to-and-fro vertigo lasting minutes to hours and followed or accompanied by headache and sensitivity to light and noise. However, even in adults, only 70% of patients with vestibular migraine present with headache. In children, its presentation varies and might be atypical, particularly in those younger than 10 years (Langhagen et al. 2016). Discrete central ocular motor signs (saccadic pursuit) are commonly observed between attacks. In contrast to headache, vertigo does not respond well to acute therapy with non-steroidal analgesics or triptans. Prophylactic treatment is indicated for frequent (≥3/month) or severe (e.g., vomiting, unable to get up and attend school) attacks. Topiramate has also been shown to prevent basilar migraine in children. Empirical evidence, as well as inference from the responses of classic migraine to treatment in adults, suggests that propranolol, metoprolol, valproic acid, amitriptyline, and flunarizine are effective therapies.

5.1.3.3 Acute Unilateral Vestibular Loss (UVL) in Children

In children, viral labyrinthitis is often associated with hearing loss (Wiener-Vacher 2008). Hearing impairment does not occur in typical UVL, which is probably caused by reactivated herpes infection. Both forms occur in children. Treatment depends on the etiology. In the acute stage, vestibular suppressants are useful (dimenhydrinate, 1–2 mg/kg); however, they should not be given for more than 3 days. Mobilization should start as soon as possible to support recalibration of the vestibular system by mechanisms of central compensation (adaptation of cerebellar and brainstem circuits). Infectious labyrinthitis and serous labyrinthitis in otitis of the middle ear are treated by antibiotics if bacterial infection is present. In non-infectious neuritis, steroids can improve vestibular recovery.

> Head trauma causes acute unilateral vestibular deficits in children more often compared to adults. This is often the case in trauma with petrous bone fractures. The symptoms are like in acute unilateral failure in the context of any other origin. One should keep in mind that the most common type of vertigo occurring after head trauma is BPPV.

Endolymphatic hydrops and Menière's disease in children are more often secondary, e.g., occurring after viral labyrinthitis, than in adults. Overall, Menière's disease is rare in children. Prophylactic treatment with betahistine dihydrochloride (1–2 mg/kg/day) is possible if required.

5.1.3.4 Vestibular Paroxysmia and Perilymphatic Fistula in Children

These patients present with short attacks of rotatory or to-and-fro vertigo (seconds). Attacks of vestibular paroxysmia can be elicited by hyperventilation in some patients (Lehnen et al. 2015). The response to treatment is important for the diagnosis. Patients usually respond well to low-dose treatment with carbamazepine. Therapy can be reduced once the patient has been free of attacks for 4 weeks.

Typical attacks in perilymphatic fistula last for seconds and also occur with pressure changes, e.g., in airplanes, but also during coughing and sneezing or lifting. A fistula is more common in children than in adults (Balatsouras et al. 2007). For diagnostic purposes, attacks can be provoked by Valsalva maneuvre; pressure to the tragus of the ear can also be helpful. Outer fistula occurs if the round or oval window in the middle ear ruptures; inner fistula occurs if the bone layer on the anterior canal to the middle cranial fossa is dehiscent (spontaneously or post-traumatically). High-resolution computed tomography of the mastoid bone can reveal labyrinth dysplasia and superior canal dehiscence. In most cases, the avoidance of provoking factors is sufficient therapy. Surgery is rarely necessary, only when the children cannot perform seriously any sports, e.g., rolling, moving fast (in posterior canal dehiscence).

5.1.3.5 Central Vestibular Vertigo in Children

Central vestibular disturbances are caused by lesions in the brainstem (in vestibular nuclei, ocular-motor nuclei, medial longitudinal fascicle, reticular formation, and midbrain tegmentum) and in the cerebellum (flocculus and nodulus). Supratentorial lesions (thalamus and cortex) rarely cause rotatory vertigo, but affected patients can present with dizziness and deviation of the subjective vertical (Jahn 2016). Clinical examination of ocular motor deficits allows the topographic diagnosis of central vestibular syndromes. Tumors of the brainstem and the cerebellum can cause vertigo in children. Magnetic resonance imaging should be performed if the clinical examination reveals central ocular motor signs. Therapy corresponds to the etiology (vascular, inflammatory, degenerative, or neoplastic). Sometimes symptomatic treatment is useful to reduce oscillopsia and postural imbalance (e.g., aminopyridines in downbeat nystagmus syndrome). Physical therapy with posture and gait training is recommended in chronic syndromes (e.g., cerebellar ataxia).

Episodic Ataxia Type 2

This is a rare autosomal dominant inherited disorder with mutation in the CACNA1A gene, coding for a subunit of the P/Q calcium channel (Strupp et al. 2007). The mutation causes Purkinje cell dysfunction in the cerebellum. Patients present with attacks of gait imbalance, dysarthria, and vertigo provoked by physical exertion. Attacks last for minutes to hours. Between attacks, clinical examination shows a cerebellar syndrome with ocular motor signs (e.g., downbeat nystagmus) and gait ataxia. The syndrome usually manifests in childhood. Therapy includes medical prophylaxis by either acetazolamide or 4-aminopyridine (Strupp et al. 2017).

Hereditary Vertigo Syndromes and Malformations

Several congenital syndromes are associated with vestibular dysfunction. Malformations of the labyrinth occur after embryopathic infections (e.g., rubella, cytomegalovirus). Mondini's dysplasia and CHARGE syndrome (coloboma, heart malformation, choanal atresia, retardation, genital hypoplasia, ear abnormality) cause dysplasia of inner ear structures. These patients often present with bilateral vestibular failure. Other structural abnormalities include children with an enlarged vestibular aqueduct (EVAS syndrome) who most often are born with a severe SNHL or deafness.

Rare syndromes with specific vestibular deficits include familial vestibular areflexia and familial vestibulopathy. In neurofibromatosis 2, vestibular symptoms are caused by vestibular schwannoma. In Usher syndrome (type 1), progressive loss of hearing and vision go along with the vestibular deficits. Friedreich ataxia, mitochondrial syndromes, and metabolic disorders (Refsum's disease) can affect vestibular function. Therapy depends on the specific disorder and is usually symptomatic. The effect size of such treatment differs widely between affected subjects (Jahn 2016).

Functional Dizziness in Children

Functional complaints are common in adolescence. In young adults, "phobic postural vertigo" is the most common diagnosis (Jahn 2016; Jahn et al. 2015b). Patients with functional syndromes present with chronic dizziness and normal findings on clinical examination and vestibular testing. Usually, the symptoms worsen in certain situations (e.g., at school, in department stores). Treatment consists of

- Complete diagnostic workup to re-assure both patients and parents
- De-sensibilization and recommendation of physical activity
- Behavioral therapy in the more severe cases

Motion Sickness in Children

Babies and children younger than 2 years are resistant to motion sickness; in contrast, children between 4 and 10 years of age are more susceptible than adults (Huppert et al. 2019). The cause of motion sickness is thought to be an intersensory conflict between the visual and vestibular systems. Children younger than 2 years do not use the visual system for dynamic spatial orientation. If vegetative signs, nausea, and vomiting are part of the motion sickness, it is most likely provoked by low frequency vertical oscillations (0.2 Hz). Head movements and lack of visual control worsen the symptoms (Cha et al. 2021). It can be prevented by visual control (looking out of the car) and avoidance of head movements. Drug prophylaxis is indicated in symptomatic cases, e.g., dimenhydrinate (1–2 mg/kg), 1 h before exposure to such situations. This dosage can be repeated every 6 h.

Important aspects regarding dizziness in elderly age are as follows:

- The entire diagnostic spectrum known in other age groups is present
- Benign paroxysmal positional vertigo (BPPV) is most common
- Sensory deficits (bilateral vestibular loss) and central vertigo are also common
- Functional (phobic) disorders and vestibular migraine are less common than in young patients, and

other factors have a greater role in elderly patients (peripheral neuropathy, orthostatic dysregulation).

5.2 Dizziness and Vertigo in the Aging Population

Figure 5.2 and Table 5.4 summarize common causes of vertigo and dizziness in elderly age. Table 5.5 summarizes common causes of gait abnormalities in elderly age.

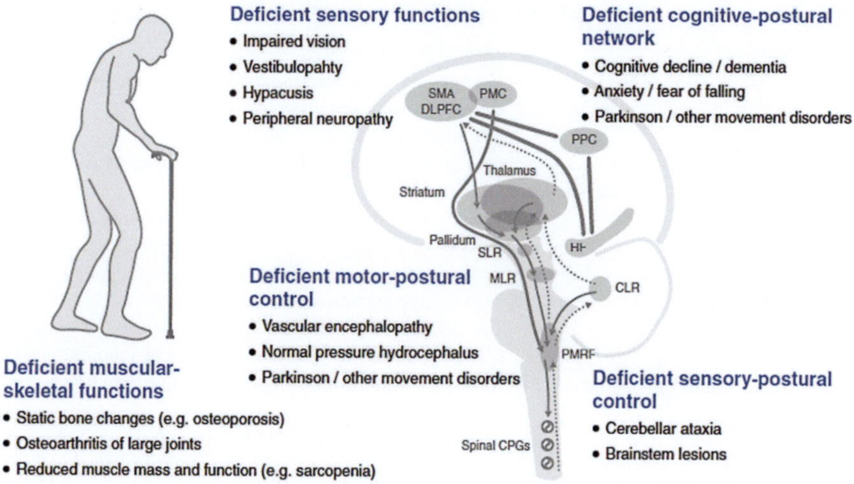

Fig. 5.2 Dizziness and imbalance in elderly age

Table 5.4 Common causes of vertigo and dizziness in the elderly

Disorder	Typical presentation
Benign Paroxysmal Positional Vertigo (BPPV)	Attacks (5–60 s) when changing head position; symptomatic in the morning; Treatment with specific physical maneuvers
Orthostatic Dizziness	Dizziness when standing up from a lying / sitting position, sometimes related to medication; Treatment with regulation of blood pressure
Menière's Disease	Vertigo episodes (minutes—hours) with ear pressure, tinnitus, hypacusis; progressive hearing loss; Treatment e.g., with Betahistine
Bilateral Vestibulopathy	Dizziness and gait instability while walking, in darkness and on uneven ground, oscillopsia; Treatment with balance training
Central vertigo and dizziness	Sustained dizziness with neurological signs (e.g., ocular motor, coordination, motor); focal signs in stroke patients, generalized signs with cerebral small vessel disease or neurodegeneration (e.g., cerebellar ataxia); Treatment of underlying disorder, balance training, symptomatic drug treatment

Relevant factors relate to one of the following four domains (Table 5.6):

- Biomechanics and joint kinematics
- Sensorimotor and neural control of balance and gait
- Cardio-pulmonary dysregulation
- Cognition, anxiety, and fear of falling

Table 5.5 Common causes of gait abnormalities in the elderly

Impairment	Typical presentation
Sensory deficits (neuropathy, Bilateral Vestibulopathy, reduced vision)	Complaints while walking, in particular with reduced light and on uneven ground; Treatment with stance- and gait-training
Neurodegeneration (Parkinsonian syndromes, Cerebellar Ataxia, Dementia)	Gait disorder with additional motor, coordinative, cognitive signs; Treatment of the underlying disorder, training of stance and gait
Normal Pressure Hydrocephalus and Vascular Encephalopathy	Hypokinetic gait disorder with subcortical dementia and bladder dysfunction, cognitive decline; Treatment with regulation of blood pressure (vascular encephalopathy) or ventriculo-peritoneal shunting
Fear of falling and intoxication (alcohol, drugs)	Slow gait with support-seeking arm movements, avoidance behavior; Treatment with reduction of medication (in case of intoxication and side effects), behavioral training, training of stance and gait

Table 5.6 Domains of balance impairments in elderly subjects

Causes	Examples
Biomechanics and kinematics	• Osteoarthritis of large joints • Degeneration of the vertebral column • Static changes in osteoporosis • Reduced muscle function due to sarcopenia and deficit of training
Sensorimotor and neural control	• Reduced vision (eye and brain) • Peripheral neuropathy / radiculopathy (e.g., vitamine B12 deficiency) • Vestibulopathy / auditory deficits • Disorders of central motor control (cerebellum, basal ganglia, brainstem, connectivity) – Parkinsonian syndromes – Cerebellar syndromes – Vascular encephalopathy – Normal pressure hydrocephalus
Cognition and anxiety	• Dementia/impairment of executive functions • Spatial orientation deficits • Fall related psychological concerns with fear of falling

Further, the individual exposure to risk affects mobility and frequency of falls (Skelton et al. 2004). Major areas to look at in this context are sensory functions, central movement control, cognition, and anxiety.

In contrast to anatomical structures, vestibular function remains rather stable in elderly age. Tests for vestibulo-ocular reflex (VOR) function like caloric irrigation and video head impulses show very little changes with age (Peterka and Black 1990a, b; Peterka et al. 1990a, b). A decline in VOR function starts above the age of 75 years. Interestingly, some responses like eye torsion and medium latency leg muscle activity in response to galvanic vestibular stimulation increase with age up to the sixth decade and decline thereafter, a finding that was explained by central compensatory mechanisms counterbalancing the peripheral structural loss (Jahn et al. 2003b, a).

In patients over 75 years of age, dizziness is the most common presenting symptom (Furman et al. 2010). The 1-year prevalence for significant dizziness that prompts a visit to the doctor and restricts activities of everyday life in persons older than 60 is 20%; in those older than 70, it is 30%, and in those older than 80, 50% (Jonsson et al. 2004). In the context of the population-based KORA-Age study in the Augsburg area (Germany), dizziness was identified as a crucial factor for an impaired quality of life and reduced participation in age-appropriate activities in elderly persons (Mueller et al. 2014b, a).

Most of the old patients with long-term dizziness also experience gait abnormalities. Balance problems that are often described as dizziness and gait instability are very common in the elderly (Strobl et al. 2023).

With increasing age, cerebral control of walking increases and, simultaneously, the central sensory interaction is often impaired (Zwergal et al. 2012). In some forms of dementia, for example, in the early phases of vascular and frontotemporal dementia and Alzheimer's disease, gait disorders and falls occur as simultaneous symptoms of cognitive decline. Studies have shown that an impaired gait can be a predictor of dementia at a later stage (Beauchet et al. 2016; Gassner et al. 2017). The concept of "motoric cognitive risk syndrome"' (MCR syndrome) has been proposed for elderly patients with subjective cognitive impairment and slow gait (>1 standard deviation under the age-specific mean). Persons with MCR syndrome are at risk of developing a degenerative form of dementia (Verghese et al. 2014). Dual task performance provides an insight into the functional locomotor-cognitive reserves of an elderly person (Freiberger 2018). This ability is often impaired before obvious cognitive or locomotor deficits manifest. Dual task paradigms also help in the differential diagnosis. Fall related psychological concerns ("Fear of falling") is a prime concern of many elderly patients with unstable gait (Payette et al. 2016). The prevalence of this fear has been reported in different studies between 21% and 85% (Reelick et al. 2009). Compared with controls of the same age, fearful patients walk more slowly. The fall related psychological concern is associated with anxiety disorders and depression and substantially impairs a person's quality of life (van Haastregt et al. 2008). Because of fall related psychological concerns, increasing avoidance behaviors reduce the confidence in one's own balance even further, so that symptoms increase in the sense of a downward spiral.

The medical history of older patients with dizziness and vertigo should capture factors that may escape attention in the clinical exam. It is important to find out, which medications a patient is taking. Sedating drugs for vertigo (cinnarizine, dimenhydrinate) are in general not suited for long-term therapy.

5.2.1 Diagnostic Findings and Differential Diagnosis

While taking a history, one should ask about falls and about the situations where such falls occurred. Distinction needs to be made between whether a patient almost fell ("near-fall") or did fall. Dizziness and unsteady gait indicate (combinations of) specific deficits that might include deficits in peripheral and central sensory functions (visual, vestibular, somatosensory), musculoskeletal insufficiencies (sarcopenia, arthritis), deficits in cognitive postural control, and anxiety (Jahn et al. 2015a).

In the normal aging process, the speed of walking continually decreases; after the age of 60, it reduces by about 1% every year (Jahn et al. 2010). Although slowing down in elderly age has many causes that interrelated in multifarious and complicated ways, walking speed has been found to be a very meaningful parameter in assessing old persons' health (Studenski et al. 2011). It is even regarded as the sixth vital sign (Wuehr et al. 2020). If a person spontaneously walks slower than 0.6 m/s, he or she will mostly require help. By contrast, virtually all persons who walk faster than 1 m/s will be independent (Jahn et al. 2015a). Among elderly patients who present to doctors, the following causes for gait disorders are particularly common:

- Sensory deficits (e.g., polyneuropathy)
- Neurodegeneration (e.g., Parkinson's disease, cerebellar ataxia)
- Cognitive deficits and anxiety (e.g., dementia, fear of falls)

In addition, antalgic (e.g., osteoarthritis of the knee) and paretic (e.g., disc herniation) gait disorders account for a large proportion of patients in general practice, orthopedic surgery, and neurology (Snijders et al. 2007). Important aspects in association with unsteady gait in elderly age include the function of the sensory systems, cognitive reserve, and locomotor reserve (Verghese et al. 2013). All these aspects must be covered by the diagnostic workup.

Perception of verticality can be measured as subjective visual (SVV), subjective haptic (SHV), and subjective postural vertical (SPV) (Nolan et al. 2022). Aging processes influence the SPV during standing and sitting. With increasing age, the perceived vertical shifts backwards, i.e., it is tilted in the posterior direction and the risk of falls in the sagittal plane rises (Bergmann et al. 2020). The reduced sensitivity may reflect an age-related decline of vestibular and somatosensory functions. These sensory systems are involved in creating and updating the central representation of verticality (Jahn et al. 2017).

5.2.2 Time Course and Therapy

Concerning acute dizziness, e.g., in acute unilateral vestibulopathy (UVL) or stroke, it must be considered that vestibular compensation slows down in elderly age. Whereas a 40-year-elderly person needs about 65 days for full recovery, a 60-year-elderly needs 140, and a 80-year-elderly 300 days for recovery from static and dynamic vestibular deficits on average. In other words, the time for compensation doubles every 20 years (Jahn et al. 2019b). Compensation and recovery are reachable but need much more effort.

Elderly subjects should receive VRT with combined eye-head exercises, active training for posture, and gait for substitution as well as counselling to prevent a functional transition of the complaints. Due to the slowing of compensation, they need longer periods of training and an adapted program for home training.

Most syndromes in the elderly, however, cause chronic problems, due to the disorders and factors mentioned and displayed above. It is of utmost importance to identify components of the individual syndrome. These components are treated as described in the respective chapters.

5.2.3 Risks and Pitfalls

The sensory control of walking is important especially in the context of slow walking and is less relevant in fast, automatic walking (Jahn et al. 2015a). Gait variability after sensory deficits increases particularly for slow walking (Wuehr et al. 2013). In parallel, the risk of falls increases which correlates with gait variability (Schulein et al. 2017).

Alterations of balance and gait performance with advanced age reflect both physiological aging of multiple body functions and structures, and the accumulation of pathologies. Generally, more than one factor contributes to impaired mobility and balance problems (Jahn et al. 2019a).

With aging, the interaction between brain structures for postural and locomotor control is impaired so that weighting and priority settings are altered (Jahn and Wuehr 2020). An example for such a change with aging is the cross inhibition between different sensory modalities that ensures the use of the most appropriate sensory signal for a certain task (e.g., vision instead of vestibular signals). In advanced age, this cross inhibition is reduced, and conflicts between sensory canals contribute to balance problems (Zwergal et al. 2012). Another example for impaired network interactions to executive functions is the dual task interference with postural tasks in the elderly (Bridenbaugh and Kressig 2015).

> Studies have shown that a partial cause of the fear of falling in elderly age may be the interaction between the sensory systems, for example, between the visual and vestibular systems. Affected persons receive too much feedback about their multisensory environment. Physical training therapy can reduce the fear of falling in the short term.

References

Abu-Arafeh I, Russell G (1995) Paroxysmal vertigo as a migraine equivalent in children: a population-based study. Cephalalgia 15(1):22–25

Balatsouras DG, Kaberos A, Assimakopoulos D et al (2007) Etiology of vertigo in children. Int J Pediatr Otorhinolaryngol 71(3):487–494

Beauchet O, Allali G, Annweiler C et al (2016) Association of motoric cognitive risk syndrome with brain volumes: results from the GAIT study. J Gerontol A Biol Sci Med Sci 71:1081. https://doi.org/10.1093/gerona/glw012

van de Berg R, Widdershoven J, Bisdorff A et al (2021) Vestibular migraine of childhood and recurrent vertigo of childhood: diagnostic criteria consensus document of the Committee for the Classification of Vestibular Disorders of the Barany Society and the International Headache Society. J Vestib Res 31(1):1–9. https://doi.org/10.3233/VES-200003

Bergmann J, Bardins S, Prawitz C et al (2020) Perception of postural verticality in roll and pitch while sitting and standing in healthy subjects. Neurosci Lett 730:135055. https://doi.org/10.1016/j.neulet.2020.135055

Bridenbaugh SA, Kressig RW (2015) Motor cognitive dual tasking: early detection of gait impairment, fall risk and cognitive decline. Z Gerontol Geriatr 48(1):15–21. https://doi.org/10.1007/s00391-014-0845-0

Cha YH, Golding J, Keshavarz B et al (2021) Motion sickness diagnostic criteria: consensus document of the classification committee of the Barany society. J Vestib Res 31:327. https://doi.org/10.3233/VES-200005

Fife TD, Tusa RJ, Furman JM et al (2000) Assessment: vestibular testing techniques in adults and children: report of the Therapeutics and Technology Assessment Subcommittee of the American Academy of Neurology. Neurology 55(10):1431–1441

Filippopulos FM, Albers L, Straube A et al (2017) Vertigo and dizziness in adolescents: risk factors and their population attributable risk. PLoS One 12(11):e0187819. https://doi.org/10.1371/journal.pone.0187819

Freiberger E (2018) Cognition and mobility: the influence of the brain on gait. Der Internist 59(4):316–325. https://doi.org/10.1007/s00108-018-0391-8

Furman JM, Raz Y, Whitney SL (2010) Geriatric vestibulopathy assessment and management. Curr Opin Otolaryngol Head Neck Surg 18(5):386–391. https://doi.org/10.1097/MOO.0b013e32833ce5a6

Gassner H, Marxreiter F, Steib S et al (2017) Gait and cognition in Parkinson's disease: cognitive impairment is inadequately reflected by gait performance during dual task. Front Neurol 8:550. https://doi.org/10.3389/fneur.2017.00550

van Haastregt JC, Zijlstra GA, van Rossum E et al (2008) Feelings of anxiety and symptoms of depression in community-living older persons who avoid activity for fear of falling. Am J Geriatr Psychiatry 16(3):186–193. https://doi.org/10.1097/JGP.0b013e3181591c1e

Huppert D, Grill E, Brandt T (2019) Survey of motion sickness susceptibility in children and adolescents aged 3 months to 18 years. J Neurol 266(Suppl 1):65–73. https://doi.org/10.1007/s00415-019-09333-w

Jahn K (2016) Vertigo and dizziness in children. Handb Clin Neurol 137:353–363. https://doi.org/10.1016/B978-0-444-63437-5.00025-X

Jahn K, Wuehr M (2020) Postural control mechanisms in mammals, including humans. In: Fritzsch B, Straka H (eds) The senses: a comprehensive reference, vol 6. Elsevier, Academic, Amsterdam, pp 344–370

Jahn K, Naessl A, Schneider E et al (2003a) Inverse U-shaped curve for age dependency of torsional eye movement responses to galvanic vestibular stimulation. Brain 126(Pt 7):1579–1589

Jahn K, Naessl A, Strupp M et al (2003b) Torsional eye movement responses to monaural and binaural galvanic vestibular stimulation: side-to-side asymmetries. Ann N Y Acad Sci 1004:485–489

Jahn K, Zwergal A, Schniepp R (2010) Gait disturbances in old age: classification, diagnosis, and treatment from a neurological perspective. Dtsch Arztebl Int 107(17):306–315

Jahn K, Kressig RW, Bridenbaugh SA et al (2015a) Dizziness and unstable gait in old age: etiology, diagnosis and treatment. Deutsches Arzteblatt Int 112(23):387–393. https://doi.org/10.3238/arztebl.2015.0387

Jahn K, Langhagen T, Heinen F (2015b) Vertigo and dizziness in children. Curr Opin Neurol 28(1):78–82. https://doi.org/10.1097/WCO.0000000000000157

Jahn K, Muller F, Koenig E et al (2017) Rehabilitation of verticality perception using a new training method. J Neurol 264(Suppl 1):26–27. https://doi.org/10.1007/s00415-017-8435-x

Jahn K, Freiberger E, Eskofier BM et al (2019a) Balance and mobility in geriatric patients : assessment and treatment of neurological aspects. Z Gerontol Geriatr 52(4):316–323. https://doi.org/10.1007/s00391-019-01561-z

Jahn K, Lopez C, Zwergal A et al (2019b) Vestibular rehabilitation therapy in Europe: chances and challenges. J Neurol 266(Suppl 1):9–10. https://doi.org/10.1007/s00415-019-09368-z

Jonsson R, Sixt E, Landahl S et al (2004) Prevalence of dizziness and vertigo in an urban elderly population. J Vestib Res 14(1):47–52

Langhagen T, Landgraf MN, Huppert D et al (2016) Vestibular migraine in children and adolescents. Curr Pain Headache Rep 20(12):67. https://doi.org/10.1007/s11916-016-0600-x

Lehnen N, Langhagen T, Heinen F et al (2015) Vestibular paroxysmia in children: a treatable cause of short vertigo attacks. Dev Med Child Neurol 57(4):393–396. https://doi.org/10.1111/dmcn.12563

Mueller M, Strobl R, Jahn K et al (2014a) Impact of vertigo and dizziness on self-perceived participation and autonomy in older adults: results from the KORA-age study. Qual Life Res 23(8):2301–2308. https://doi.org/10.1007/s11136-014-0684-x

Mueller M, Strobl R, Jahn K et al (2014b) Burden of disability attributable to vertigo and dizziness in the aged: results from the KORA-age study. Eur J Pub Health 24(5):802–807. https://doi.org/10.1093/eurpub/ckt171

Nolan J, Jacques A, Godecke E et al (2022) Post-stroke lateropulsion terminology: pushing for agreement amongst experts. Ann Phys Rehabil Med 65(6):101684. https://doi.org/10.1016/j.rehabilitation.2022.101684

Payette MC, Belanger C, Leveille V et al (2016) Fall-related psychological concerns and anxiety among community-dwelling older adults: systematic review and meta-analysis. PLoS One 11(4):e0152848. https://doi.org/10.1371/journal.pone.0152848

Peterka RJ, Black FO (1990a) Age-related changes in human posture control: motor coordination tests. J Vestib Res 1(1):87–96

Peterka RJ, Black FO (1990b) Age-related changes in human posture control: sensory organization tests. J Vestib Res 1(1):73–85

Peterka RJ, Black FO, Schoenhoff MB (1990a) Age-related changes in human vestibulo-ocular and optokinetic reflexes: pseudorandom rotation tests. J Vestib Res 1(1):61–71

Peterka RJ, Black FO, Schoenhoff MB (1990b) Age-related changes in human vestibulo-ocular reflexes: sinusoidal rotation and caloric tests. J Vestib Res 1(1):49–59

Reelick MF, van Iersel MB, Kessels RP et al (2009) The influence of fear of falling on gait and balance in older people. Age Ageing 38(4):435–440. https://doi.org/10.1093/ageing/afp066

Schulein S, Barth J, Rampp A et al (2017) Instrumented gait analysis: a measure of gait improvement by a wheeled walker in hospitalized geriatric patients. J Neuroeng Rehabil 14(1):18. https://doi.org/10.1186/s12984-017-0228-z

Skelton DA, Becker C, Lamb SE, Close JCT, Zijlstra W, Yardley L, Todd CJ (2004) Prevention of Falls Network Europe: a thematic network aimed at introducing good practice in effective falls prevention across Europe. Eur J Ageing. 1(1):89–94. https://doi.org/10.1007/s10433-004-0008-z. Epub 2004 Nov 4. PMID: 28794706; PMCID: PMC5547692

Snijders AH, van de Warrenburg BP, Giladi N et al (2007) Neurological gait disorders in elderly people: clinical approach and classification. Lancet Neurol 6(1):63–74. https://doi.org/10.1016/S1474-4422(06)70678-0

Strobl R, Harajli S, Huppert D, Zwergal A, Grill E (2023) Impact of episodic and chronic vestibular disorders on health-related quality of life and functioning-results from the DizzyReg patient registry. Qual Life Res. 32(6):1717–1726. https://doi.org/10.1007/s11136-023-03345-w. Epub 2023 Jan 25. PMID: 36698042

Strupp M, Zwergal A, Brandt T (2007) Episodic ataxia type 2. Neurotherapeutics 4(2):267–273

Strupp M, Teufel J, Zwergal A et al (2017) Aminopyridines for the treatment of neurologic disorders. Neurol Clin Pract 7(1):65–76. https://doi.org/10.1212/CPJ.0000000000000321

Studenski S, Perera S, Patel K et al (2011) Gait speed and survival in older adults. JAMA 305(1):50–58. https://doi.org/10.1001/jama.2010.1923

Verghese J, Wang C, Lipton RB et al (2013) Motoric cognitive risk syndrome and the risk of dementia. J Gerontol A Biol Sci Med Sci 68(4):412–418. https://doi.org/10.1093/gerona/gls191

Verghese J, Annweiler C, Ayers E et al (2014) Motoric cognitive risk syndrome: multicountry prevalence and dementia risk. Neurology 83(8):718–726. https://doi.org/10.1212/WNL.0000000000000717

Wiener-Vacher SR (2008) Vestibular disorders in children. Int J Audiol 47(9):578–583. https://doi.org/10.1080/14992020802334358

Wuehr M, Schniepp R, Ilmberger J et al (2013) Speed-dependent temporospatial gait variability and long-range correlations in cerebellar ataxia. Gait Posture 37(2):214–218. https://doi.org/10.1016/j.gaitpost.2012.07.003

Wuehr M, Huppert A, Schenkel F et al (2020) Independent domains of daily mobility in patients with neurological gait disorders. J Neurol 267(Suppl 1):292–300. https://doi.org/10.1007/s00415-020-09893-2

Yang J, Liu Y, Zhang Q et al (2023) Editorial: vestibular disorders in children. Front Neurol 14:1142504. https://doi.org/10.3389/fneur.2023.1142504

Zwergal A, Linn J, Xiong G et al (2012) Aging of human supraspinal locomotor and postural control in fMRI. Neurobiol Aging 33(6):1073–1084

Dizziness in Cerebral Disorders

6

6.1 Dizziness in Head Trauma and After Concussion

After head trauma/concussion, dizziness is one of the most frequent symptoms within the first 72 h (Ernst et al. 2005). It is primarily based on a labyrinthine concussion (e.g., in sports-related concussion-SRC-, Mucha et al. 2018), but the prognosis is dependent on the central vestibular impairment (as in post-concussion syndrome-PCS and/or mild traumatic brain injury—MTBI) (Dwyer and Katz 2018; Katz et al. 2015).

6.1.1 Diagnostic Findings and Differential Diagnosis

After the acute trauma (e.g., blunt head trauma, sports-related concussion = SRC), the patients should undergo a vestibular/ocular motor screening procedure to identify peripheral/central impairment (e.g., spontaneous/head-shake nystagmus, pathological HIT, gaze/smooth pursuit testing) and a possible overlap with MTBI/whiplash-associated disorder (= WAD; McKeithan et al. 2019; Kontos et al. 2017, Ekvall Hansson et al. 2006) as soon as possible. This is important to plan extended diagnostics (e.g., complete neuro-otological workup) (Basta et al. 2005, 2007) and therapy/rehabilitation. Special emphasis should be put on blast exposed patients (usually military personal) because they are most likely patients with subsequent MTBI/neuropsychiatric disorders (e.g., PTSD) and a delayed recovery (Akin et al. 2017; Denby et al. 2020). Neuroimaging is indicated with mor GCS severity and/or red flag clinical findings (MRI and/or HR-CT of the petrous bone) should reliably exclude central vestibular pathology and/or intracochlear hemorrhage/microfractures of the otic capsule, particularly in children (Ernst et al. 2005; Ellis et al. 2015; Clement 2019). One rare, but existing problem is the exacerbation of a hitherto unknown/clinically silent SCDS upon the head impact (Fig. 6.1).

A. Ernst et al., *Vestibular Therapy and Rehabilitation*,
https://doi.org/10.1007/978-3-031-64318-7_6

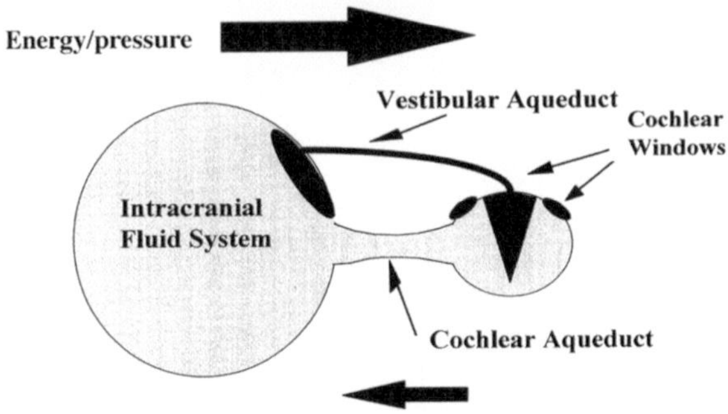

Fig. 6.1 Upon concussion/impact, a pressure wave passes from the CSF space to the inner ear through its connecting pathways (cochlear/vestibular aqueduct) and impairs the cochlear/vestibular receptor cells

6.1.2 Time Course and Therapy

The head trauma and/or concussion should be treated adequately based on GCS assessment and neuropsychological testing. There is no "standard"therapy available yet, but the pharmacological approaches are aimed at providing neuroprotection and prevent cerebral hypertension/CSF pressure increase (for review, see Ng and Lee 2019).

Specific medication for the dizziness complaints should only be given in case of intralabyrinthine hemorrhage with UVL and include systemic steroids (Ernst et al. 2005) and/or symptomatic antiemetics (Basta et al. 2017). No sedatives should be given, but after at least 48 h, PT should start (Alsalaheen et al. 2010). Patients with a prolonged recovery should be treated also with symptomatic pharmacotherapy (Lercher and Camiolo Reddy 2014). Apart from severe head trauma and complete otolith loss, most of the patients recover within 6 months by means of PT and/or specific training (e.g., NFT) (Ernst et al. 2007; Basta et al. 2008). However, those with additional PCS and/or WAD can benefit from VRT, but long-term benefits cannot always be found (Kleffelgaard et al. 2019; Sinnott et al. 2019).

There is no uniform physiological time window for recovery after concussion, but there is evidence that the physiological dysfunction (of the brain and the vestibular system) can outlast that of clinical recovery, particularly in those with risk factors as described below (Kamins et al. 2017). Predictors for a poor outcome of the VRT in posttraumatic vertigo is the parallel occurrence of central vestibular impairment (Gimmon et al. 2017), elderly age (King 2014) and—well documented for SRC (Morgan et al. 2015)—personal/family history of mood disorders, psychiatric illness, migraine, delayed onset of PCS, previous head trauma(s).

6.1.3 Risk and Pitfalls

Patients can suffer from dizziness, imbalance, and restricted mobility after stroke for several reasons. These include (1) specific vestibular lesions and lesions in balance networks (brainstem, cerebellum), (2) widespread brain lesions with a more general dizziness (microangiopathic changes), and (3) functional dizziness after stroke due to the fear to get a next stroke and a pathological increased of perception of the own physiological balance control.

6.2 Dizziness After Stroke/Cerebral Ischemia

6.2.1 Diagnostic Findings and Differential Diagnosis

Ischemic or haemorrhagic strokes directly affecting vestibular structures and networks often have a relatively benign prognosis with improvements of deficits over days to weeks (Schuhbeck et al. 2022). However, affected patients need intensive rehabilitation and training. The paradigmatic vestibular stroke is Wallenberg's syndrome due to an ischemic lesion in the postero-lateral medulla oblongata (Fig. 6.2). Other parts of the central balance network can also be affected: midline cerebellum, brainstem tegmentum, lateral thalamus (Zwergal et al. 2020). Cortical lesions in the vestibular and multisensory regions (temporo-parietal junction) rarely cause longstanding balance problems.

Many patients with widespread lesions due to microangiopathic changes report dizziness as their major complaint. This is not caused by specific vestibular involvement, but by a general network insufficiency that causes preferentially problems with cognition and balance. Clinical presentation is very similar in multiple

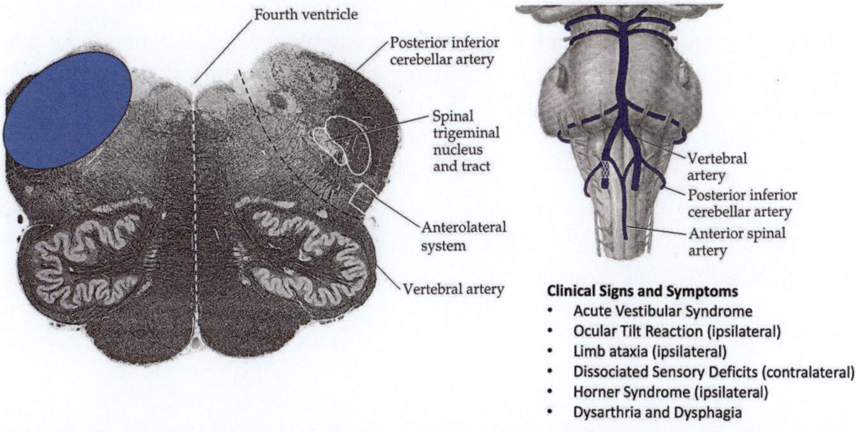

Fig. 6.2 Wallenberg's syndrome: Clinical presentation and site of lesion

sclerosis with multiple lesions and in normal pressure hydrocephalus (Jahn et al. 2015; Wuehr et al. 2020).

Functional dizziness with fear of falling or depression often develops after stroke. For differentiation of lesional causes, the clinical examination and review of imaging findings are essential. It is crucial to identify the functional component of a post-stroke syndrome as treatment differs from lesional dizziness (Schuhbeck et al. 2022).

The most important tools for differentiation of different forms of post-stroke dizziness are clinical examination and brain imaging (MRI) to correlate findings and complaints.

6.2.2 Time Course and Therapy

Deficits after vestibular strokes (dorsolateral medulla = Wallenberg's syndrome, midline cerebellum) improve over days to weeks. They rarely cause chronic problems. Patients need early mobilization and vestibular rehabilitation therapy to speed up recovery and to prevent secondary functional dizziness (Meldrum et al. 2020; Whitney et al. 2020).

Patients with vascular encephalopathy (widespread microangiopathic changes) have chronic problems. When arterial hypertension, nicotine consumption, and diabetes are not well controlled, symptoms and deficits get worse over time. These patients require continuous balance training including dual-task paradigms to improve mobility, balance, and cognition.

In functional dizziness, the general recommendation to increase physical activity is more important than specific (vestibular) rehabilitation training (Tschan et al. 2013).

6.2.3 Risks and Pitfalls

Patients after stroke have a high risk for further vascular events. It is important that they follow the recommendations including prophylactic drug therapy, lifestyle modifications, and physical activity. The risk to develop a functional dizziness is high if disorder, treatment, and prognosis are not well explained to the patient.

> Patients with early phase Parkinson's disease, normal pressure hydrocephalus, dementia, and cerebellar ataxia often present to dizziness units before the diagnosis was met (Schlick et al. 2016).

6.3 Dizziness in Neurodegenerative and Inflammatory Brain Disorders

6.3.1 Diagnostic Findings and Differential Diagnosis

A neurological examination of dizzy patients must be done in all cases where the presentation suggests an underlying brain disease. This is the case with ocular motor abnormalities, severe postural imbalance, and cognitive deficits (Schniepp et al. 2021). The diagnosis of neurodegenerative disorders is often made in tertiary dizziness units. The same is true for chronic inflammatory diseases. The by far most common one is multiple sclerosis. In primary progressive disease, patients often present with spastic-ataxic gait and recurrent falls.

Among Parkinson's patients and beside dizziness, the ones with idiopathic disease present most often with asymmetric symptoms, tremor, hypomimia, and bradykinesia. Among the atypical syndromes, progressive supranuclear palsy (PSP) is the most common in dizziness units (Zwergal et al. 2013). These patients report on recurrent falls and show vertical > horizontal saccade slowing on ocular motor testing. Postural reflexes are severely affected. VOR function, by definition, is unimpaired. All Parkinson's patients need one standard brain MRI.

In cerebellar ataxia, diagnosis can easily be made by testing ocular motor, balance, and coordinative functions. Patients show saccadic pursuit, disturbed suppression of the VOR, dysmetric pointing tests, and postural imbalance, sometimes with 3 Hz sway (Schniepp et al. 2022).

In demented patients, findings on balance tests range from normal to severely affected. The key findings come from cognitive testing with reduced attention and difficulties with problem solving in subcortical dementia (normal pressure hydrocephalus and vascular encephalopathy) and disturbed spatial orientation and cortical functions (e.g., aphasia) in cortical dementia like Alzheimer's disease.

Clinical presentation in multiple sclerosis and other inflammatory diseases can be very divers, dependent on the distribution of lesions.

6.3.2 Time Course and Therapy

All disorders in this chapter show a chronic progressive cause due to neurodegeneration or vasculopathy. Concerning therapy, patients need the specific therapy for their disorder (e.g., L-Dopa drug treatment in Parkinson's disease). Besides this, all patients with central movement disorders all need physical therapy to improve gait and balance. It is well known that patients with Parkinson's disease benefit from vestibular training as well. In Parkinson's disease balance, training is crucial. For cerebellar ataxia, there is some evidence as well that training can improve balance and general well-being. In dementia, mobility and walking can slow down cognitive decline. Patients with multiple sclerosis also benefit from physical therapy including specific balance training.

6.3.3 Risks and Pitfalls

Making the diagnosis early on can be difficult, in particular in environments not experienced with the disorders. The clinical course will often help. It is therefore recommended to reassess unclear cases after 3–6 months. Expert neurological opinion should be involved. However, for most of the neurodegenerative disorders, a causal therapy is not available. Symptomatic treatments are nowadays effective and should be provided.

6.4 Dizziness and Epilepsy

Vestibular epileptic spells are rare (Tarnutzer et al. 2015). However, some forms of seizures, with temporal, hippocampal, or frontal origin, start with a dizzy aura that is followed by motor symptoms and/or by reduced consciousness. In chronic epilepsy, some patients develop dizziness as a side effect of medication (carbamazepine, oxcarbazepine, and many more), due to the decline of cognition or in relation to anxiety and fear of falling.

References

Akin FW, Murnane OD, Hall CD et al (2017) Vestibular consequences of mild traumatic brain injury and blast exposure: a review. Brain Inj 31(9):1188–1194. https://doi.org/10.1080/02699052.2017.1288928

Alsalaheen BA, Mucha A, Morris LO et al (2010) Vestibular rehabilitation for dizziness and balance disorders after concussion. J Neurol Phys Ther 34(2):87–93. https://doi.org/10.1097/NPT.0b013e3181dde568

Basta D, Todt I, Scherer H et al (2005) Postural control in otolith disorders. Hum Mov Sci 24(2):268–279. https://doi.org/10.1016/j.humov.2005.04.002

Basta D, Clarke A, Ernst A et al (2007) Stance performance under different sensorimotor conditions in patients with post-traumatic otolith disorders. J Vestib Res 17(1):25–31

Basta D, Singbartl F, Todt I et al (2008) Vestibular rehabilitation by auditory feedback in otolith disorders. Gait Posture 28(3):397–404. https://doi.org/10.1016/j.gaitpost.2008.01.006

Basta D, Borsellino L, Ernst A (2017) Antivertiginous drug therapy does not hinder the efficacy of individualized vibrotactile neurofeedback training for vestibular rehabilitation—a randomized trial. Int J Rehabil Res 40(4):333–338. https://doi.org/10.1097/MRR.0000000000000245

Clement MO (2019) Imaging of brain trauma. Radiol Clin North Am 57(4):733–744. https://doi.org/10.1016/j.rcl.2019.02.008

Denby E, Murphy D, Busuttil W et al (2020) Neuropsychiatric outcomes in UK military veterans with mild traumatic brain injury and vestibular dysfunction. J Head Trauma Rehabil 35(1):57–65. https://doi.org/10.1097/HTR.0000000000000468

Dwyer B, Katz DI (2018) Postconcussion syndrome. Handb Clin Neurol 158:163–178. https://doi.org/10.1016/B978-0-444-63954-7.00017-3

Ekvall Hansson E, Mansson NO, Ringsberg KA et al (2006) Dizziness among patients with whiplash-associated disorder: a randomized controlled trial. J Rehabil Med 38(6):387–390. https://doi.org/10.1080/16501970600768992

Ellis MJ, Leiter J, Hall T et al (2015) Neuroimaging findings in pediatric sports-related concussion. J Neurosurg Pediatr 16(3):241–247. https://doi.org/10.3171/2015.1.PEDS14510

Ernst A, Basta D, Seidl RO et al (2005) Management of posttraumatic vertigo. Otolaryngol Head Neck Surg 132(4):554–558. https://doi.org/10.1016/j.otohns.2004.09.034

Ernst A, Singbartl F, Basta D et al (2007) Short-term rehabilitation of patients with posttraumatic otolith disorders by auditory feedback training: a pilot study. J Vestib Res 17(2–3):137–144

Gimmon Y, Millar J, Pak R et al (2017) Central not peripheral vestibular processing impairs gait coordination. Exp Brain Res 235(11):3345–3355. https://doi.org/10.1007/s00221-017-5061-x

Jahn K, Kressig RW, Bridenbaugh SA et al (2015) Dizziness and unstable gait in old age: etiology, diagnosis and treatment. Deutsches Arzteblatt Int 112(23):387–393. https://doi.org/10.3238/arztebl.2015.0387

Kamins J, Bigler E, Covassin T et al (2017) What is the physiological time to recovery after concussion? A systematic review. Br J Sports Med 51(12):935–940. https://doi.org/10.1136/bjsports-2016-097464

Katz DI, Cohen SI, Alexander MP (2015) Mild traumatic brain injury. Handb Clin Neurol 127:131–156. https://doi.org/10.1016/B978-0-444-52892-6.00009-X

King NS (2014) A systematic review of age and gender factors in prolonged post-concussion symptoms after mild head injury. Brain Inj 28(13–14):1639–1645. https://doi.org/10.3109/02699052.2014.954271

Kleffelgaard I, Soberg HL, Tamber AL et al (2019) The effects of vestibular rehabilitation on dizziness and balance problems in patients after traumatic brain injury: a randomized controlled trial. Clin Rehabil 33(1):74–84. https://doi.org/10.1177/0269215518791274

Kontos AP, Deitrick JM, Collins MW et al (2017) Review of vestibular and oculomotor screening and concussion rehabilitation. J Athl Train 52(3):256–261. https://doi.org/10.4085/1062-6050-51.11.05

Lercher K, Camiolo Reddy C (2014) Treating prolonged symptoms of mild traumatic brain injury: neuropharmacology. Prog Neurol Surg 28:139–148. https://doi.org/10.1159/000358771

McKeithan L, Hibshman N, Yengo-Kahn AM et al (2019) Sport-related concussion: evaluation, treatment, and future directions. Med Sci (Basel) 7(3). https://doi.org/10.3390/medsci7030044

Meldrum D, Burrows L, Cakrt O et al (2020) Vestibular rehabilitation in Europe: a survey of clinical and research practice. J Neurol 267(Suppl 1):24–35. https://doi.org/10.1007/s00415-020-10228-4

Morgan P, McDonald R, McGinley J (2015) Perceived cause, environmental factors, and consequences of falls in adults with cerebral palsy: a preliminary mixed methods study. Rehabil Res Pract 2015:196395. https://doi.org/10.1155/2015/196395

Mucha A, Fedor S, DeMarco D (2018) Vestibular dysfunction and concussion. Handb Clin Neurol 158:135–144. https://doi.org/10.1016/B978-0-444-63954-7.00014-8

Ng SY, Lee AYW (2019) Traumatic brain injuries: pathophysiology and potential therapeutic targets. Front Cell Neurosci 13:528. https://doi.org/10.3389/fncel.2019.00528

Schlick C, Schniepp R, Loidl V et al (2016) Falls and fear of falling in vertigo and balance disorders: a controlled cross-sectional study. J Vestib Res 25(5–6):241–251. https://doi.org/10.3233/VES-150564

Schniepp R, Huppert A, Decker J et al (2021) Fall prediction in neurological gait disorders: differential contributions from clinical assessment, gait analysis, and daily-life mobility monitoring. J Neurol 268(9):3421–3434. https://doi.org/10.1007/s00415-021-10504-x

Schniepp R, Huppert A, Decker J et al (2022) Multimodal mobility assessment predicts fall frequency and severity in cerebellar ataxia. Cerebellum 22:85. https://doi.org/10.1007/s12311-021-01365-1

Schuhbeck F, Strobl R, Conrad J et al (2022) Determinants of functioning and health-related quality of life after vestibular stroke. Front Neurol 13:957283. https://doi.org/10.3389/fneur.2022.957283

Sinnott AM, Elbin RJ, Collins MW et al (2019) Persistent vestibular-ocular impairment following concussion in adolescents. J Sci Med Sport 22(12):1292–1297. https://doi.org/10.1016/j.jsams.2019.08.004

Tarnutzer AA, Lee SH, Robinson KA et al (2015) Clinical and electrographic findings in epileptic vertigo and dizziness: a systematic review. Neurology 84(15):1595–1604. https://doi.org/10.1212/WNL.0000000000001474

Tschan R, Best C, Wiltink J et al (2013) Persistence of symptoms in primary somatoform vertigo and dizziness: a disorder "lost" in health care? J Nerv Ment Dis 201(4):328–333. https://doi.org/10.1097/NMD.0b013e318288e2ad

Whitney SL, Sparto PJ, Furman JM (2020) Vestibular rehabilitation and factors that can affect outcome. Semin Neurol 40(1):165–172. https://doi.org/10.1055/s-0039-3402062

Wuehr M, Huppert A, Schenkel F et al (2020) Independent domains of daily mobility in patients with neurological gait disorders. J Neurol 267(Suppl 1):292–300. https://doi.org/10.1007/s00415-020-09893-2

Zwergal A, la Fougere C, Lorenzl S et al (2013) Functional disturbance of the locomotor network in progressive supranuclear palsy. Neurology 80(7):634–641. https://doi.org/10.1212/WNL.0b013e318281cc43

Zwergal A, Mohwald K, Salazar Lopez E et al (2020) A prospective analysis of lesion-symptom relationships in acute vestibular and ocular motor stroke. Front Neurol 11:822. https://doi.org/10.3389/fneur.2020.00822

Dizziness in Other Medical Condition

7

7.1 Dizziness in Psychiatric and Psychosomatic Conditions

Functional dizziness accounts for up to one-third of patients presenting to the large tertiary dizziness clinics. This is due to the chronic character of the complaints and to the high degree of individual restriction caused by the symptoms.

7.1.1 Diagnostic Findings and Differential Diagnosis

Functional dizziness is the most common diagnosis in young adults between 18 and 40 years (Strupp 2005). The diagnosis can be made by the typical history (e.g., symptoms also at rest, fluctuations with aggravation in certain environments, worsening over the day, sensitivity to moving visual scenes) and the typical findings on clinical examination (e.g., normal finding or findings not explaining the symptoms, postural imbalance in simple tasks that improves in more difficult tasks) (Brandt et al. 1997). A presumed pathophysiological concept is depicted in Fig. 7.1. There is a high comorbidity with psychiatric and psychosomatic disorders (Lahmann et al. 2015). Psychiatric disorders (e.g., depression) are often suspected on clinical presentation. It depends on the clinical presentation if counselling the patient is sufficient or if psychological and psychiatric therapeutic support is needed. Differential diagnoses for chronic complaints are (a combination with) sensory deficits and early phases of neurodegeneration.

7.1.2 Time Course and Therapy

For treatment of functional dizziness, counselling and education are the most important interventions (Brandt et al. 2010). As soon as the patient can understand and

A. Ernst et al., *Vestibular Therapy and Rehabilitation*, https://doi.org/10.1007/978-3-031-64318-7_7

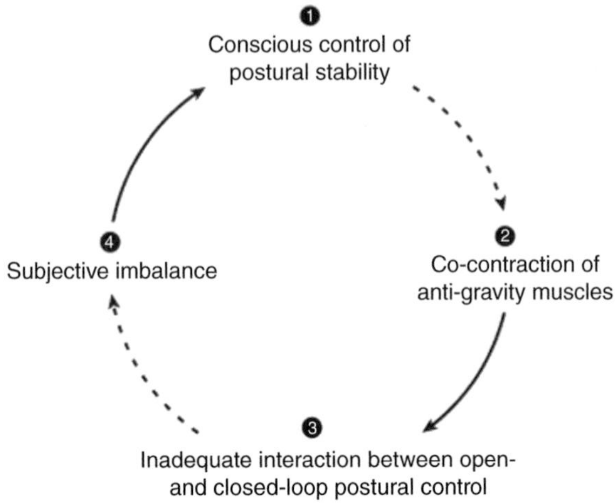

Fig. 7.1 Pathophysiology of functional dizziness and anxiety-related symptoms (Wuehr et al. 2013)

accept the explanation of the experienced dizziness, further chances to successfully treat the disorder are high. Most patients become better after presentation to centers which know about the disorder (Brandt and Dieterich 2020). Treatment can be supported by multimodal approaches combining psychological and physical treatment elements (Tschan et al. 2012). Medication is sometimes needed. Selective serotonin reuptake inhibitors (SSRIs) are most often used. They only have an effect if combined with counselling. Psychiatric comorbidities should be treated as well, but often require consultation of the psychiatrist.

7.1.3 Risks and Pitfalls

Most patients do not like to get driven in a psychiatric corner. There is a high risk to "lose the patient" that gets the impression that nothing was found and therefore a psychological/psychiatric explanation is thought. It is important to explain, that functional dizziness is a well-defined disorder that can accordingly be treated. Another pitfall is the attribution of the patient's complaints to functional dizziness in organic disorders. This can best be prevented by careful history-taking, complete clinical examination, and a good knowledge of potential differential diagnoses.

7.2 Dizziness with Peripheral Neuropathy

Discussion on peripheral neuropathy had also been included in Chap. 5 as it is often part of the syndrome presenting with dizziness and gait instability in elderly people (Jahn et al. 2015). As peripheral neuropathy is very common in advanced age, it remains difficult to determine if the neuropathy really explains the symptoms. A typical clinical presentation is like BVL. Patients report on gait instability that becomes worse with reduced visual control (eyes closed, darkness) and on uneven ground. In contrast to BVL, patients also report numbness and tingling sensation in their feet. On clinical examination, the neuropathy is suspected when the Romberg test shows pathological findings (worsening with eyes closed), tendon reflexes are absent at least at the distal legs (Achilles tendon reflex), and proprioception is reduced.

Peripheral neuropathy is most often caused by diabetes or chronic alcohol consumption. Other causes include vitamin B12 deficiency, hematological, rheumatological, and nephrological diseases. Treatment should include balance training with active standing and walking, performed as specifically as possible adapted to the deficit.

7.3 Dizziness After Cochlear Implantation

7.3.1 Occurrence and Etiology

Hearing loss is the most common sensory deficit of all. It affects about one-third of people above 65 years of age. Nowadays, patients with severe hearing loss or deafness are commonly implanted with a cochlear implant (CI) uni- or bilaterally. CI attempts to replace the function of hair cells by stimulating spiral ganglion cells of the auditory nerve electrically in response to sound. While the effects of CI surgery on hearing thresholds and communication are well studied, less attention has been given to its effects on vestibular function.

Even today, CI surgery frequently affects the vestibular apparatus, which is in close anatomical proximity to the auditory system.

In the early 1990s, approximately 60% of the patients suffered from vertigo after cochlear implant surgery (van den Broek et al. 1993). The symptoms were mainly related to the surgical trauma while inserting the electrode array into the cochlea. Thus, the loss of inner ear fluids, perilymphatic fistulae, and the occurrence of a benign paroxysmal positional vertigo have been described. The portion of patients with long-lasting vestibular problems dropped within the last years to 10%–20% (higher values with increasing age) due to the development of soft surgery techniques (Hansel et al. 2018). However, the vestibular dysfunction is currently still the most common side effect of cochlear implantation. Due to the risk of a vestibular receptor damage, a sequential implantation is always recommended for bilaterally CI candidates. The sequential implantation gives the opportunity to easily compensate a possible unilateral vestibular damage postoperatively and to estimate the risk of a second surgery for the quality of life.

The statistically significant most frequently damaged vestibular sensor is the saccule followed by the semicircular canals and the utricle (Table 7.1). Thus, the vertigo after cochlear implantation is mainly related to a saccular disorder.

The saccule seems to be the main target since it is located very close to the cochlear implant insertion side. The induced histological damage upon an electrode insertion is shown in Fig. 7.2. The example indicates a distortion of the saccular membrane which could occur during high-pressure changes upon electrode insertion. High cochlear pressure changes were measured in different models of CI surgery (Todt et al. 2014) and seem to play an important role also for hearing preservation in CI patients with residual low frequency hearing. These high-pressure changes are able to damage cochlear and vestibular structures as previously described for noise exposures. An electrode insertion into the scala vestibuli instead of the scala tympani could amplify such damages (Tien and Linthicum Jr. 2002).

Table 7.1 Overview about the percentage of function loss in specific vestibular sensors upon cochlear implantation in relation to the surgical electrode insertion approach (c = insertion via cochleostomy, rw = round window insertion)

Semicircular canal dysfunction	Saccular dysfunction	Utricular dysfunction	Surgical approach	Reference
43	50		c	Todt et al. (2008)
9	13		rw	Todt et al. (2008)
6	67		c	Basta et al. (2008b)
58	50		c	Krause et al. (2009b)
32			c	Krause et al. (2009a)
	82		c	Licameli et al. (2009)
39	51		c	Jacot et al. (2009)
6	31		rw	Melvin et al. (2009)
50	86		c	Krause et al. (2010)
6	23		rw	Wagner et al. (2010)
	61	87	c	Xu et al. (2015)
73	62		rw	Louza et al. (2015)
72	59		rw	Robard et al. (2015)
18	76		rw	Meli et al. (2016)
93	42	37	rw	Chen et al. (2016)
38	46		rw	Nordfalk et al. (2016b)
20	58		rw	Nordfalk et al. (2016a)
14	44		c	Nordfalk et al. (2016a)
16	16	19	rw	Sosna et al. (2019)
	12	5	rw	Dagkiran et al. (2019)
21			rw	Stuermer et al. (2019)
11	16	9	rw	Tsukada and Usami (2021)

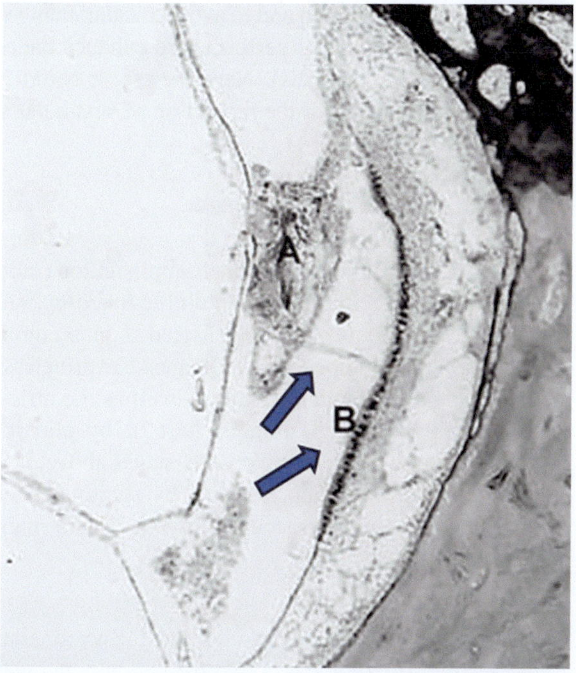

Fig. 7.2 Saccular membrane distortion upon cochlear implant electrode insertion. (**A**) Distorted saccular membrane. (**B**) Saccular sensory epithelium, arrows indicate pathological movements of the saccular membrane (after Tien and Linthicum Jr. 2002)

Beside the direct trauma, caused by the electrode insertion, other mechanisms could play a role for the generation of vertigo and dizziness after cochlear implantation. An acute serous labyrinthitis due to cochleostomy, a specific foreign body reaction which can develop a labyrinthitis, the development of an endolymphatic hydrops or the electrical co-stimulation from the implant itself is under discussion. The latter was shown to occur in patients stimulated by high current level with the lowest thresholds on apical electrodes (Basta et al. 2008b; Coordes et al. 2012).

7.3.2 Prevention

Some research was performed within the last years to prevent the occurrence of vestibular disorders after cochlear implantation. The first approach was to perform soft surgery with an electrode insertion via the round window without performing a cochleostomy. Especially the occurrence of otolith disorders was reduced by changing the surgical approach to approximately one-third for the utricle and to one half for the saccule (Table 7.1). However, the frequency of SCC disorders was not affected. Another important development was the reduction of pressure changes applied to vestibular and residual cochlear hair cells by lowering the electrode insertion speed. This technique was extensively investigated and resulted in the recommendation to insert as slow as possible (appr. 100 μm/s) without any additional movements (Todt et al. 2014, 2016). Furthermore, electrode design was adapted for a very atraumatic insertion and to avoid a scalar change (Todt et al. 2017). The latter developments were mainly performed to enhance the prevention of residual natural hearing (cochlear hair cells). Nevertheless, it could be assumed that these techniques are also helpful for the protection of vestibular structures and function.

7.3.3 Diagnostic Procedures

Long-lasting dizziness after cochlear implantation (more than 2–3 weeks) should be analyzed with a specific focus on otolithic function. Since unilateral loss of semicircular function is frequently compensated soon, an otolith disorder (even unilateral) is much harder to compensate at all ages. Nevertheless, the function of all semicircular canals on the implanted side as well as the utricular function should be analyzed by the video head impulse test or by eliciting ocular vestibular evoked myogenic potentials, respectively. As stated above, it is mandatory to test the saccular function on the implanted side by eliciting cervical vestibular evoked myogenic potentials since a saccular disorder is the main reason for dizziness after cochlear implantation.

> It could be very helpful to compare the postoperative results with preoperative testing. Hearing loss is frequently combined with vestibular dysfunctions since vestibular and cochlear structures are tightly connected by similar liquids and common cavities. A vestibular function loss could be possibly already present before a cochlear implant surgery even without complaints (compensated). All postoperative changes in vestibular function are more likely responsible for the occurrence of vertigo after cochlear implant surgery.

Postoperative vertigo should be related to an electrical co-stimulation of the vestibular nerve if it starts just after or during the activation of the cochlear implant function (first fitting of the sound processor). The co-stimulation could be objectified by measuring the EMG of neck muscles (sternocleidomastoid muscle, trapezoid muscle) upon stimulation. A co-stimulation mainly affects the inferior part of the vestibular nerve which connects the saccule with the vestibular brainstem nuclei. The EMG activation could be triggered by sound application to the CI-processor (Coordes et al. 2012) or by increasing stimulation values.

7.3.4 Therapy

A changed cochlear implant fitting could resolve the problem if a sound-induced vertigo was detected. The apical electrodes, which are mostly responsible for the electrical co-stimulation, should be switched into the bipolar mode (for a more local stimulation) or the stimulation current should be reduced. Sometimes, it is necessary to switch off some of the electrodes.

In rare cases (appr. 1% of all implantations), a perilymphatic fistula (leakage of perilymph at the oval or round window) could be associated with chronic dizziness after cochlear implantation. It was shown that a transtympanic resealing of the electrode insertion side (round window) by the positioning of a new series of fascia patches leads to a symptom relief in most patients (Karimi et al. 2017).

The treatment effort of physical therapy depends largely on the specific vestibular disorder which was induced by the electrode insertion.

Unilateral SCC function loss is frequently successfully treatable with conventional VRT focusing on the stimulation of the vestibular ocular reflex through head movements. However, in cases of otolith dysfunction, it seems that physical therapy targeting postural control and orientation of the head and body may also beneficial, as these appear to be the primary functions of the otolith organs. However, otolith disorders frequently require more intense technical approaches.

Fortunately, such technical treatment options for otolith disorders improved over the last decade markedly. Especially neurofeedback techniques seem to be most effective for the compensation of the diminished input. Furthermore, walking conditions (under different sensory conditions) should be implemented in a rehabilitation program since patients with otolith disorders frequently report instability during walking. A successful neurofeedback training in stance and gait conditions was first reported for auditory feedback (Basta et al. 2008a). A more effective option is the vibrotactile neurofeedback training since it is much more individualized and intuitive (Basta et al. 2011). In brief, it starts with a measurement of postural control during a mixture of daily-life stance and gait tasks under different sensory conditions. Tasks with pathological sway are selected for the rehabilitation training. During the training, patients receive a vibrotactile stimulus if their sway is outside a given limit (based on normative values and patients' performance). Large improvements were described after a daily 10 min training for 10 days. Such a neurofeedback training is also effective in some other vestibular diseases (Basta et al. 2017; Basta et al. 2011) but nearly mandatory for chronic otolith disorders.

7.4 Dizziness in Ophthalmology, Cardiology, and Orthopedics

Different medical conditions can lead to dizziness and vertigo without directly interfering with the vestibular receptor and system, respectively. Therefore, the patient's individual history is of utmost importance to direct the therapist and to enable proper diagnostics, apart from neurotological testing. In this chapter, the most important pathologies which can cause vertigo and dizziness will be mentioned, but no extensive procedures (neither diagnostic nor therapeutic) can be addressed.

7.4.1 Diagnostic Findings and Differential Diagnosis

Cardiovascular disorders (arterial hypertension, cardiac arrhythmia, neuro-cardiogenic syncope, postural orthostatic tachycardia syndrome—POTS-, orthostatic hypotension). Usually, the patients complain of a sudden onset of dizziness which can lead to unconsciousness. A specialized workup with blood pressure monitoring, cardiological and tilt table testing is advised.

Ophthalmic disorders (aberration disorders, disorders of binocular stereo vision, disturbed eyeball motility). Ocular dizziness is very unspecific and requires a diagnostic workup of central and peripheral ocular motility, including the optic and all ocular motor nerves (namely Nn. II, III, IV, VI), myositis of the intraorbital muscles, and supranuclear eyeball motility disorders (e.g., downbeat nystagmus, INO). An easy test to differentiate between ocular/ non-ocular dizziness is to ask the patients if symptoms disappear when they close their eyes.

Neuro-orthopedic disorders (spinal concussion/ whiplash, postsurgical complications, stenosis of the spinal canal). Except for chronic conditions (e.g., stenosis of the spinal canal), all other disorders have an acute onset after the external trigger (trauma/ surgery). Most patients complain of pain, a limitation of the CROM and an increase in trunk sway which can be recorded by mobile posturography. In all those conditions, neuroimaging (MRI/MRA) should be performed (Fig. 7.3).

7.4.2 Time Course and Therapy

The time course of those disorders is highly variable as is therapy (dependent on the medical disciplines involved) so that no guidelines exist.

Acute onset

↓

Neurological/MRI/manual medicine diagnostics (CROM)

↓

Pain management, passive mobilization, manual therapy

↓

Home training for postural muscles

Fig. 7.3 PT in neuro-orthopedic disorders with acute onset (e.g., whiplash injury, post-surgery of the cervical spine) (MRI: magnetic resonance imaging of the cervical spine; CROM: determination of the cervical range of motion)

7.4.3 Risks and Pitfalls

The elderly patients with several disorders and an extensive drug intake pose a risk of being underdiagnosed since the different medical conditions and drug intakes (polypharmacy!) frequently bear the risk of creating dizziness. A sequence of tests and involvement of medical disciplines is time-consuming, but necessary to adequately correlate the type of dizziness with the responsible medical condition (or drug) (Fig. 7.4).

1

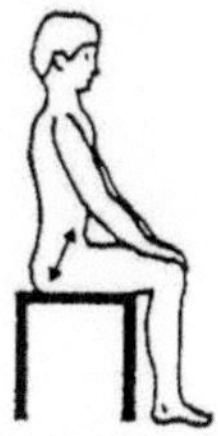

Balanced body position- sitting upright:
Sway into an upright sitting position, tense up your abdominal and posterior muscles, bring your shoulders together backwards while breathing deeply, slowly without pressing (correct sitting position, breathing techniques and body self-perception).

2

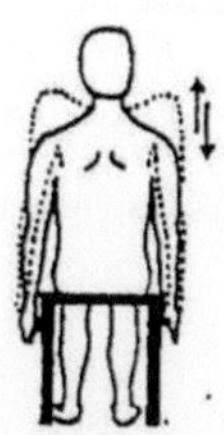

Basic body tension while sitting:
Press feet on the ground with a shoulder distance in between, tense up your abdominal and posterior muscles (i.e., basic body tension), pull your shoulders actively down and your head up (spine stretching), then pull your shoulders up, hold them for 5 s and circle them back and forward (mobilisation and strengthening of the shoulder-neck muscles).

3

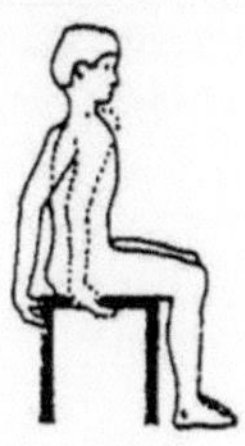

Building up body tension:
Press your shoulders actively together backwards and down, hold them for 5 s, then push them up and forward (direction of your nose) while pulling up your head and keep your abdominal and posterior muscles tensed up (stretching and strengthening of the breast and shoulder muscles).

4

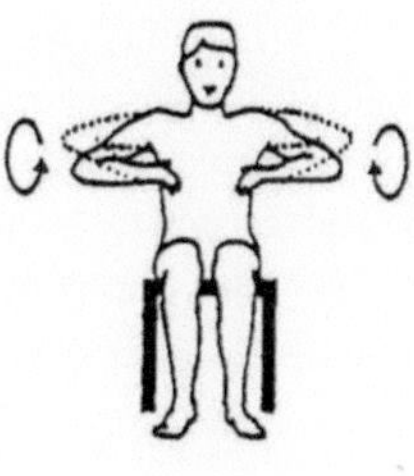

Basic body tension while sitting:
Put your thumbs under your axilla and circle with your arms in large extensions back- and forward (mobilisation and strengthening of the shoulder-neck muscles).

5

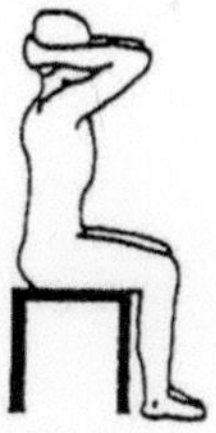

Basic body tension while sitting:
Put your hands together behind your head and press slowly and gently your head against your hands (it must be comfortable, not painful!), then release the tension slowly (do the exercise about 10x) (stabilisation of the cervical spine, strengthening of the neck muscles).

Fig. 7.4 Home exercises for the cervical/ thoracal spine

6

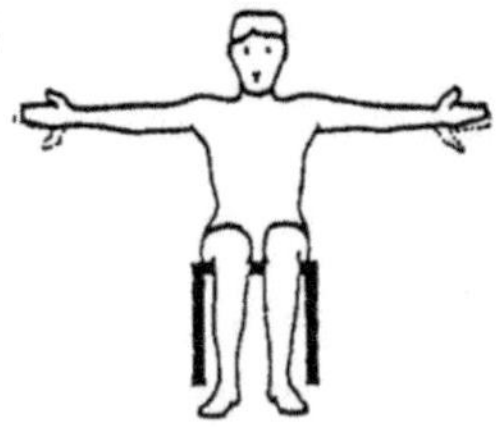

Basic body tension while sitting:
Stretch your arms to the side and turn them back- and forward as much as possible (for about 20 s) and lift your head up (mobilisation of the shoulder girdle, stabilisation of the neck and shoulder muscles).

7

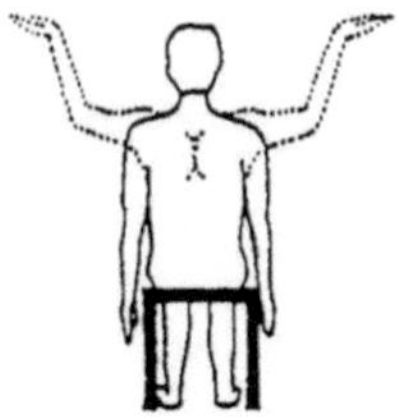

Basic body tension while sitting:
Put your arms rectangularly up, pull your elbows back and press with your hands up (against a virtual resistance) (strengthening of the neck, shoulder and spinal muscles)

8

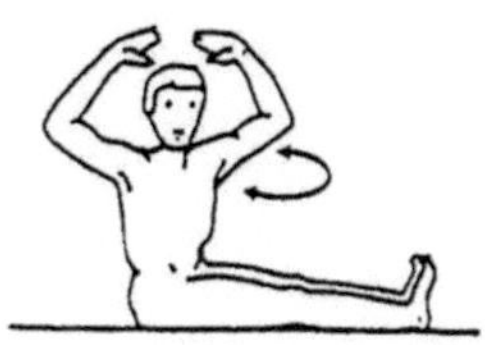

Stretch seat:
Keep your upper body upright and push your knees through, pull your toes towards you and lift up your head (Stretching of the posterior leg muscles, keeping body tension).

9

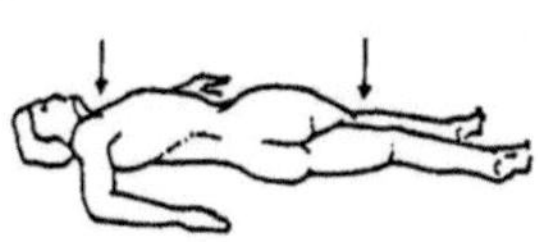

Supine position:
Arms are positioned relaxed at the side, right leg is bent and pulled over the left one, right knee touches the ground. Building up tension by pulling the right shoulder towards the ground (keeping the position for about 5 s), then do the same with the left leg (Stretching of the body muscles, mobilisation of the spine).

10

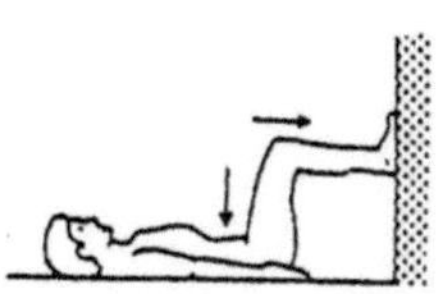

Relaxation:
In supine, push your feet against the wall so that upper and lower leg are positioned rectangularly. Build up slowly a soft pressure (comfortable!) and feel it being dispersed through the body, then release (repeat about 10x) (body self-perception and muscle activity).

Fig. 7.4 (continued)

References

Basta D, Singbartl F, Todt I, Clarke A, Ernst A (2008a) Vestibular rehabilitation by auditory feedback in otolith disorders. Gait Posture 28(3):397–404. https://doi.org/10.1016/j.gaitpost.2008.01.006

Basta D, Todt I, Goepel F, Ernst A (2008b) Loss of saccular function after cochlear implantation: the diagnostic impact of intracochlear electrically elicited vestibular evoked myogenic potentials. Audiol Neurootol 13(3):187–192. https://doi.org/10.1159/000113509

Basta D, Rossi-Izquierdo M, Soto-Varela A, Greters ME, Bittar RS, Steinhagen-Thiessen E, Eckardt R, Harada T, Goto F, Ogawa K, Ernst A (2011) Efficacy of a vibrotactile neurofeedback training in stance and gait conditions for the treatment of balance deficits: a double-blind, placebo-controlled multicenter study. Otol Neurotol 32(9):1492–1499. https://doi.org/10.1097/MAO.0b013e31823827ec

Basta D, Borsellino L, Ernst A (2017) Antivertiginous drug therapy does not hinder the efficacy of individualized vibrotactile neurofeedback training for vestibular rehabilitation—a randomized trial. Int J Rehabil Res 40(4):333–338. https://doi.org/10.1097/MRR.0000000000000245

Brandt T, Dieterich M (2020) 'Excess anxiety' and 'less anxiety': both depend on vestibular function. Curr Opin Neurol 33(1):136–141. https://doi.org/10.1097/WCO.0000000000000771

Brandt T, Kapfhammer HP, Dieterich M (1997) "Phobic postural vertigo". A further differentiation of psychogenic vertigo conditions seems necessary. Nervenarzt 68(10):848–849

Brandt T, Huppert T, Hufner K, Zingler VC, Dieterich M, Strupp M (2010) Long-term course and relapses of vestibular and balance disorders. Restor Neurol Neurosci 28(1):69–82

van den Broek P, Huygen PL, Mens LH, Admiraal RJ, Spies T (1993) Vestibular function in cochlear implant patients. Acta Otolaryngol 113(3):263–265. https://doi.org/10.3109/00016489309135806

Chen X, Chen X, Zhang F, Qin Z (2016) Influence of cochlear implantation on vestibular function. Acta Otolaryngol 136:655–659

Coordes A, Basta D, Gotze R, Scholz S, Seidl RO, Ernst A, Todt I (2012) Sound-induced vertigo after cochlear implantation. Otol Neurotol 33(3):335–342. https://doi.org/10.1097/MAO.0b013e318245cee3

Dagkiran M, Tuncer U, Surmelioglu O, Tarkan O, Ozdemir S, Cetik F, Kiroglu M (2019) How does cochlear implantation affect five vestibular end-organ functions and dizziness? Auris Nasus Larynx 46(2):178–185. https://doi.org/10.1016/j.anl.2018.07.004

Hansel T, Gauger U, Bernhard N, Behzadi N, Romo Ventura ME, Hofmann V, Olze H, Knopke S, Todt I, Coordes A (2018) Meta-analysis of subjective complaints of vertigo and vestibular tests after cochlear implantation. Laryngoscope 128(9):2110–2123. https://doi.org/10.1002/lary.27071

Jacot E, Van Den Abbeele T, Debre HR, Wiener-Vacher SR (2009) Vestibular impairments pre- and post-cochlear implant in children. Int J Pediatr Otorhinolaryngol 73:209–217

Jahn K, Kressig RW, Bridenbaugh SA, Brandt T, Schniepp R (2015) Dizziness and unstable gait in old age: etiology, diagnosis and treatment. Deutsches Arzteblatt Int 112(23):387–393. https://doi.org/10.3238/arztebl.2015.0387

Karimi D, Mittmann P, Ernst A, Todt I (2017) Surgical treatment of vertigo in cochlear implantees by electrode resealing. Acta Otolaryngol 137(10):1031–1034. https://doi.org/10.1080/00016489.2017.1331045

Krause E, Louza JPR, Hempel J-M, Wechtenbruch J, Rader T, Gürkov R (2009a) Effect of cochlear implantation on horizontal semicircular canal function. Eur Arch Otorhinolaryngol. 266(6):811–817. https://doi.org/10.1007/s00405-008-0815-5.

Krause E, Wechtenbruch J, Rader T, Berghaus A, Gürkov R (2009b) Impaired fixation suppression is a risk factor for vertigo after cochlear implantation. J Laryngol Otol. 123(8):845–850. https://doi.org/10.1017/S0022215109004812.

Krause E, Louza JPR, Wechtenbruch J, Gürkov R (2010) Influence of cochlear implantation on peripheral vestibular receptor function. Otolaryngol Head Neck Surg 142(6):809–813. https://doi.org/10.1016/j.otohns.2010.01.017.

Lahmann C, Henningsen P, Brandt T, Strupp M, Jahn K, Dieterich M, Eckhardt-Henn A, Feuerecker R, Dinkel A, Schmid G (2015) Psychiatric comorbidity and psychosocial impairment among patients with vertigo and dizziness. J Neurol Neurosurg Psychiatry 86(3):302–308. https://doi.org/10.1136/jnnp-2014-307601

Licameli G, Zhou G, Kenna MA (2009) Disturbance of vestibular function attributable to cochlear implantation in children. Laryngoscope 119:740–745

Louza J, Mertes L, Braun T, Gurkov R, Krause E (2015) Influence of insertion depth in cochlear implantation on vertigo symptoms and vestibular function. Am J Otolaryngol 36:254–258

Meli A, Aud BM, Aud ST, Aud RG, Cristofari E (2016) Vestibular function after cochlear implant surgery. Cochlear Implants Int 17:151–157

Melvin TA, Della Santina CC, Carey JP, Migliaccio AA (2009) The effects of cochlear implantation on vestibular function. Otol Neurotol 30:87–94

Nordfalk KF, Rasmussen K, Bunne M, Jablonski GE (2016a) Deep round window insertion versus standard approach in cochlear implant surgery. Eur Arch Otorhinolaryngol 273:43–50

Nordfalk KF, Rasmussen K, Hopp E, Bunne M, Silvola JT, Jablonski GE (2016b) Insertion depth in cochlear implantation and outcome in residual hearing and vestibular function. Ear Hear 37:e129–e137

Robard L, Hitier M, Lebas C, Moreau S (2015) Vestibular function and cochlear implant. Eur Arch Otorhinolaryngol 272:523–530

Sosna M, Tacikowska G, Pietrasik K, Skarżyński H, Lorens A, Skarżyński PH (2019) Effect on vestibular function of cochlear implantation by partial deafness treatment-electro acoustic stimulation (PDT-EAS). Eur Arch Otorhinolaryngol 276(7):1951–1959. https://doi.org/10.1007/s00405-019-05425-5

Strupp M (2005) Vertigo in young adults. The ground swings—anxiety spreads. MMW Fortschr Med 147(20):55–56

Stuermer KJ, Kluenter HD, Lang-Roth R, Schwarz D, Hüttenbrink KB, Anagiotos A (2019) Preservation of Vestibular Function and Residual Hearing After Round Window Cochlear Implantation. Otol Neurotol 40(7):878–882. https://doi.org/10.1097/MAO.0000000000002257

Tien HC, Linthicum FH Jr (2002) Histopathologic changes in the vestibule after cochlear implantation. Otolaryngol Head Neck Surg 127(4):260–264. https://doi.org/10.1067/mhn.2002.128555

Todt I, Basta D, Ernst A (2008) Does the surgical approach in cochlear implantation influence the occurrence of postoperative vertigo? Otolaryngol Head Neck Surg 138:8–12

Todt I, Mittmann P, Ernst A (2014) Intracochlear fluid pressure changes related to the insertional speed of a CI electrode. Biomed Res Int 2014:507241. https://doi.org/10.1155/2014/507241

Todt I, Ernst A, Mittmann P (2016) Effects of different insertion techniques of a Cochlear implant electrode on the intracochlear pressure. Audiol Neurootol 21(1):30–37. https://doi.org/10.1159/000442041

Todt I, Mittmann M, Ernst A, Mittmann P (2017) Comparison of the effects of four different cochlear implant electrodes on intra-cochlear pressure in a model. Acta Otolaryngol 137(3):235–241. https://doi.org/10.1080/00016489.2016.1232490

Tschan R, Eckhardt-Henn A, Scheurich V, Best C, Dieterich M, Beutel M (2012) Steadfast effectiveness of a cognitive-behavioral self-management program for patients with somatoform vertigo and dizziness. Psychother Psychosom Med Psychol 62(3–4):111–119. https://doi.org/10.1055/s-0032-1304575

Tsukada K, Usami SI (2021) Vestibular Preservation After Cochlear Implantation Using the Round Window Approach. Front Neurol 27(12):656592. https://doi.org/10.3389/fneur.2021.656592.

Wagner JH, Basta D, Wagner F, Seidl RO, Ernst A, Todt I (2010) Vestibular and taste disorders after bilateral cochlear implantation. Eur Arch Otorhinolaryngol 267(12):1849–1854. https://doi.org/10.1007/s00405-010-1320-1

Wuehr M, Pradhan C, Novozhilov S, Krafczyk S, Brandt T, Jahn K, Schniepp R (2013) Inadequate interaction between open- and closed-loop postural control in phobic postural vertigo. J Neurol 260(5):1314–1323. https://doi.org/10.1007/s00415-012-6797-7

Xu XD, Zhang XT, Zhang Q, Hu J, Chen YF, Xu M (2015) Ocular and cervical vestibular-evoked myogenic potentials in children with cochlear implant. Clin Neurophysiol 126:1624–1631

Part IV

Other Therapeutic Measures and Specific Interventions in Vestibular Disorders

8 Tai Chi and Other Measures to Improve Gait and Stance Stability

The vestibular system has multiple inputs emerging from the labyrinth, the optical system, and the musculoskeletal system as the major sources. When the labyrinth is not fully functional (e.g., unilateral or bilateral vestibular loss, age-related degeneration), other additional measures can be helpful to stabilize stance and gait (apart from "classical" vestibular rehabilitation techniques). They are mostly aimed at strengthening/stabilizing/activating postural muscles and the corresponding musculoskeletal structures. However, there is no "one-fits-all" approach possible since the individual capabilities and needs of the vestibular patient must be carefully considered.

This holds true for all post-isometric exercises of the head and shoulder muscles and sports therapy, either as core-strength training for the postural muscles (primarily of the cervical and lumbar spine, e.g., KIESER training in the EU) or PILATES exercises which both have been described to improve balance in the elderly and to prevent falls (Granacher et al. 2013).

Tai Chi has been widely investigated and accepted as an add-on to VRT. It can be performed as exercises under supervision or at home, particularly by the elderly (Tsang et al. 2004; Wu et al. 2016). It has also been described as a successful post-therapy intervention when patients have plateaued in their stance and gait performance after VRT (Chow et al. 2023).

> Tai Chi is a technique dating back to the early days of Traditional Chinese Medicine (TCM) and Martial Arts. Tai Chi as a concept seeks movement and body control (by the brain) through slow (and mindful) movements "against a gentle resistance" in a continuous flow to "generate a soft inner power" (https://taichiforhealthinstitute.org/essential-tai-chi-principles-2). Balance (in the sense of upright, well-positional balance, but also as inner harmony and mental quietness) is essential in Tai Chi, especially in careful weight transference.

A. Ernst et al., *Vestibular Therapy and Rehabilitation*,
https://doi.org/10.1007/978-3-031-64318-7_8

Table 8.1 The ten principles of Tai Chi Chuan exercises (https://kung-fu.co.za/articles/10-principles-of-tai-chi-chuan)

Principle 1:
We have to be empty, agile and keep the energy at the top of our heads.
Principle 2:
We have to stretch the back and pull our chest.
Principle 3:
We have to relax our waist.
Principle 4:
We have to be able to understand and express "full" and "empty" states of our body elements.
Principle 5:
We have to relax our shoulders and elbows.
Principle 6:
We have to tactically think in a creative manner instead of using the brute force.
Principle 7:
We have to connect what is low with what is high and what is high with what is low.
Principle 8:
We have to join the inside activity with the outside one.
Principle 9:
We have to chain our movements together without interrupting the flow.
Principle 10:
We have to each the calm in any movement.

Tai Chi exercises can be learnt and applied in different ways and environments (Martial Arts Schools, Health Education Classes, even thru the internet). They should be performed regularly, even 4–8 weeks' intensive Tai Chi training only can significantly improve balance control (in the elderly) (Tsang et al. 2004). When comparing VRT with Tai Chi over a 10 weeks' period, they both were equally effective in improving gait disorders based on presbyvestibulopathy (McGibbon et al. 2005) (Table 8.1).

References

Chow K, Lei-Rivera L, Cosetti MK, Kelly JL (2023) Tai chi as an adjunctive therapy for individuals who plateau after vestibular rehabilitation. J Laryngol Otol 137(6):651–660. https://doi.org/10.1017/S0022215122001785

Granacher U, Lacroix A, Muehlbauer T, Roettger K, Gollhofer A (2013) Effects of core instability strength training on trunk muscle strength, spinal mobility, dynamic balance and functional mobility in older adults. Gerontology 59(2):105–113. https://doi.org/10.1159/000343152

McGibbon CA, Krebs DE, Parker SW, Scarborough DM, Wayne PM, Wolf SL (2005) Tai Chi and vestibular rehabilitation improve vestibulopathic gait via different neuromuscular mechanisms: preliminary report. BMC Neurol 5(1):3. https://doi.org/10.1186/1471-2377-5-3

Tsang WW, Wong VS, Fu SN, Hui-Chan CW (2004) Tai Chi improves standing balance control under reduced or conflicting sensory conditions. Arch Phys Med Rehabil 85(1):129–137. https://doi.org/10.1016/j.apmr.2003.02.002

Wu Y, MacDonald HV, Pescatello LS (2016) Evaluating exercise prescription and instructional methods used in Tai Chi studies aimed at improving balance in older adults: a systematic review. J Am Geriatr Soc 64(10):2074–2080. https://doi.org/10.1111/jgs.14242

9 Dietary Measures

There is no dietary recommendation that in general should be given to people with dizziness and balance problems. Some aspects, however, are of importance for subgroups of patients:

- **A Mediterranean diet** is known to reduce the risk for vascular events. It is in particular useful in patients after vestibular stroke and in those with increased risk for vascular complications.
- **No or not more that moderate alcohol consumption** is recommended to avoid any complications. Alcohol does not only provoke acute dizziness after ingestion due to its effects on inner ear and central cerebellar function, it also causes long-term complications. Peripheral neuropathies can be caused or aggravated by alcohol. Atrophy of the cerebellum and other parts of the brain can be caused by long-term consumption of more than one beverage per day.
- **Normal glucose levels** in the peripheral blood and normal glucose tolerance (no diabetes) are of relevance again for the function of peripheral nerves and also for the function of vestibular nerves. Manifest diabetes should be treated accordingly.
- **Substitution of vitamin B12 if necessary.** Low vitamin B12 levels are among the more common causes of peripheral neuropathy and bilateral vestibular loss.
- **Vitamin D supplementation if necessary.** Although the relation of BPPV and low vitamin D levels is not as closed as once supposed, there is an increase in BPPV at winter times.

A. Ernst et al., *Vestibular Therapy and Rehabilitation*, https://doi.org/10.1007/978-3-031-64318-7_9

10 Counselling and Coping for the Dizzy Patient

In contrast to the other sensory systems, e.g., vision, hearing, or light touch, people are much less aware of the normal working mode of their vestibular or balance sense. Education, counselling, and coping are therefore relevant to help dizzy patients to understand the nature of their symptoms and know about measures to re-calibrate the system. Knowing how the typical symptoms can be explained also helps preventing the secondary development of a functional dizziness, phobic symptoms, and avoidance behaviour.

It is in general recommended to include coping and counselling into the multi-modal therapeutic program. Specific approaches are described in the respective chapters.

A. Ernst et al., *Vestibular Therapy and Rehabilitation*,
https://doi.org/10.1007/978-3-031-64318-7_10

Index

A
Acoustic neuroma, 71–73
Activities-specific balance confidence scale, 15
Acute unilateral vestibular loss (UVL) in children, 88
Acute vestibular syndrome (AVS), 60, 77
Adaptation, 8
Adaptation exercises, 9
Analgesics, 23
Anterior canal BPPV, 57
Audiological testing, 21
Auditory feedback, 41–42

B
Benign paroxysmal positional vertigo (BPPV), 53–60
Benign paroxysmal vertigo of childhood, 85
Berg balance scale, 15
Bilateral vestibular loss (BVL), 62–63

C
Caloric testing, 18
Canalolithiasis, 53
Cardiovascular disorders, 114
Cardiovascular work-up, 62
Cerebellar ataxia, 103
Cervical range of motion, 24
CHARGE syndrome, 89
Children, 83
Chronic pain patient, 24
Clinical examination, 16
Cochlear implant, 109
Cochleostomy, 111
Cognitive deficits, 103
Comorbidity, 21
Compensation, 5–10
Concussion, 99–101
Counselling and coping, 125
Cupulolithiasis, 54

D
Dehiscence syndromes of the semicircular canals, 65–67
Dietary recommendation, 123
Dix-Hallpike test, 54
Dizziness handicap inventory, 15
Dizziness in childhood, 83–90
Dizziness in elderly, 90
Dynamic gait index, 15

E
Electrical co-stimulation, 111
Endolymphatic hydrops, 63–65
Epidemiology, 3–5
Episodic ataxia type 2, 89
Epley's maneuvers, 57
EVAS syndrome, 89
Exercises for acute vertigo/dizziness, 36
Exercises for balance disorders, 32
Exercises for gait disorders, 29

F
Fall efficacy scale, 16
Falls, 94
Fear of falling, 93
Feedback devices, 40
Functional dizziness, 107

A. Ernst et al., *Vestibular Therapy and Rehabilitation*,
https://doi.org/10.1007/978-3-031-64318-7

G
Gait variability, 95
Galvanic feedback, 43–44
Gaze evoked nystagmus, 20
Gufoni maneuver, 59

H
Habituation, 5–10
Habituation exercises, 10
Head-impulse test, 18
Head trauma, 99–101
Hearing loss, 63
Hereditary vertigo syndromes, 89
HINTS criteria, 77
Horizontal canal BPPV, 55–56

I
Individualized vibrotactile neurofeedback training (iNFT), 45
Ischemic or haemorrhagic strokes, 101

K
KIESER training, 121

L
Labyrinthitis, 88
Locomotor control, 95

M
Menière's disease, 63–65
Mild central ocular motor syndrome, 73
Mobile posturography, 45
Motion sickness in children, 90
Motoric cognitive risk syndrome, 93
Multiple sclerosis, 103
Musculoskeletal insufficiencies, 94

N
Neuroimaging, 21
Neurological examination, 16
Neuro-orthopedic disorders, 114
Neuropathic pain, 25
Neuro-vascular cross compression, 75

O
Occlusion of the superior SCC, 66
Ocular tilt reaction, 19
Ophthalmic disorders, 114
Oscillopsia, 62
Otoscopy, 16

P
Parkinson's patients, 103
Perception of verticality, 94
Perilymphatic fistula, 113
Perilymph fistula, 76
Peripheral neuropathy, 108
Pharmacological treatment, 23–26
Physical therapy, 26
PICA infarction, 27
PILATES exercises, 121
Polyneuropathy, 94
Post-concussion syndrome, 39
Posterior canal BPPV, 57
Post-isometric exercises, 121
Postoperative vertigo, 112
Postural imbalance, 103, 107
Presbyacusis, 63
Presbyvestibulopathy, 62
Pressure changes, 110
Progressive supranuclear palsy (PSP), 103
Psychiatric comorbidities, 108
PT in central vestibular disorders, 27–28

R
Refsum's disease, 89
Rehabilitation technology, 28–46
Root entry zone, 75

S
Saccades, 20
Screening tests, 17
Secondary prophylactic treatment, 77
Semont maneuver, 57
Skew deviation, 19
Smartphone applications, 39–40
Smooth pursuit, 18
Soft surgery, 111
Specialized VRT program, 22
Subjective haptic (SHV), 94
Subjective postural vertical (SPV), 94
Subjective visual (SVV), 94
Substitution, 9
Substitution exercises, 9

T
Tai Chi exercises, 122
Taking the history, 13
Therapy plan, 21–23

Timed-up-and-go test, 16
Transitory ischemic attacks (TIA), 77
Traumatic brain injury, 39

U
Unilateral vestibular loss, 27
Usher syndrome, 89

V
Vascular encephalopathy, 102
Vertigo symptom scale, 16
Vestibular compensation, 7, 94
Vestibular epileptic spells, 104
Vestibular function in children, 84
Vestibular implant, 63
Vestibular migraine, 64, 73–75
Vestibular migraine in children, 87–88
Vestibular paroxysmia, 75, 88–89
Vestibular strokes, 77–78, 102
Vibrotactile feedback, 44–46
Vibrotactile neurofeedback training, 113
Visual feedback, 42–43
VOR, 18, 92

W
Walking speed, 94
Wallenberg's syndrome, 77, 101
Watch & scan, 71
White noise galvanic vestibular stimulation, 63

Y
Yacovino maneouver, 59

MIX
Papier aus verantwortungsvollen Quellen
Paper from responsible sources
FSC® C105338

If you have any concerns about our products,
you can contact us on
ProductSafety@springernature.com

In case Publisher is established outside the EU,
the EU authorized representative is:
Springer Nature Customer Service Center GmbH
Europaplatz 3, 69115 Heidelberg, Germany

Printed by Libri Plureos GmbH
in Hamburg, Germany